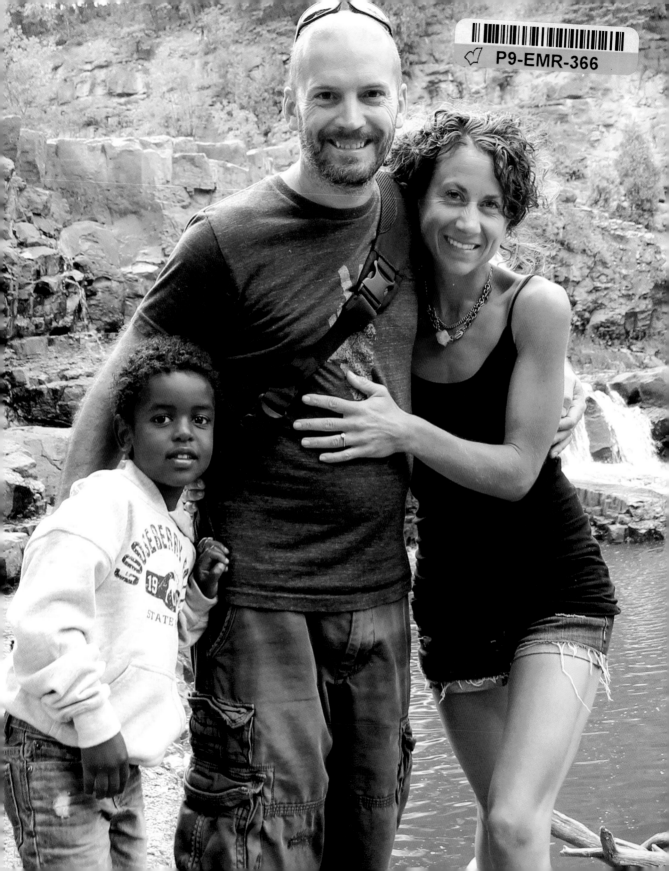

CONTENTS

chapter 1

The Failures of Modern Nutritional Guidance

"

I used to be a big fan of beer. I'm a German from Wisconsin! I brewed my own beer, and I went to beer festivals and tastings. I would eat 'fairly well' during the week and whatever I wanted on the weekends. However, over time (with my wife, Maria, setting the example) I started to realize that this lifestyle wasn't benefiting my body and health. I began to remove all grains from my diet, but I wasn't ready to let go of my beer. It wasn't until about five years ago that I realized what it was doing to me. We were with Maria's parents at their cabin, and I told Maria something was wrong with the water there. She said she felt fine and wasn't getting sick. Suddenly I realized it wasn't the water causing me to be ill; it was the beer. I am now beer-free and feel much better, plus have lost 40 pounds. I finally realized this is a lifestyle, not a diet. If a huge beer fan like me can do it, so can you!

—Craig

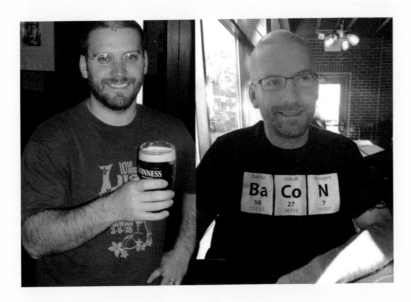

Healthcare professionals and researchers seem to view the problems and diseases that afflict us as being caused by defects in our genes or our DNA. They seem to think that all they can do is manage the symptoms of cancer, autoimmune disease, Alzheimer's disease, diabetes, and so on. In this book, we hope to shift that viewpoint so you see how perfect our bodies are. Most of the time, they do exactly what they are designed to do given the foods we eat and other inputs from our environment. Using that logic, we hope to show you that we need to change what we put into our bodies and the environments that surround us if we want to have better health. We shouldn't bandage our problems with prescription drugs; instead, we must get to the root cause of the issues.

We cover a range of topics that can help you realize your best health by changing the inputs your body receives. These inputs come from many sources, including the food you eat, your environment (light, sleep, and so on), and even what you put on your skin. Humans have evolved over hundreds of thousands of years, but our environment has drastically changed over the last couple thousand years. Our bodies are not intended to be in climate-controlled rooms that are devoid of natural sunlight year round. Humans have only recently had access to an endless supply of food, even in winter. We are not intended to consume the additives found in modern foods. In the last five decades, the number of approved food additives has skyrocketed from 800 to more than 14,000.[1] We are inundating our bodies with substances they never had to deal with before. And this problem is getting worse every day as processed foods become more and more common.

Over the last fifty years, "experts" have embraced many theories that either lack scientific backing or were brought about by corruption and manipulation. Here's a sample of some of the

INPUTS AND OUTPUTS

I was a very analytical kid. Numbers just made sense to me. I got my degree in electrical engineering and spent a lot of time in labs diagnosing problems in digital systems. Whenever there was an error in an electrical output, I would look to the inputs to determine what was causing the output error. Often, you must go back to the source—the input—of the problem and fix it so that the output is correct.

I view the body in the same way. If given the proper inputs, your body will do the right thing with them. Yes, there are true genetic disorders, but when you look at the causes of death today, the most common are metabolic diseases that can be reversed given the proper inputs.

misleading and incorrect (or partially incorrect) guidelines that we have been led to believe:

- Make sure your diet is low in fat and higher in carbohydrates because eating fat causes heart disease.
- Avoid saturated fats and cholesterol because they are bad for you and cause heart disease.
- Omit salt because it can cause high blood pressure.
- Avoid eggs and other forms of dietary cholesterol because cholesterol causes coronary artery disease.
- Use sunscreen to protect your skin because sunlight causes cancer.
- Eat whole grains because they are "heart healthy."
- Use vegetable oils and seed oils because they are "heart healthy."
- Avoid red meat and bacon because they cause cancer.
- Eat a plant-based diet because it's the healthiest diet for humans.
- Eat lots of fruit and vegetables because they are the most nutrient-dense foods.

Many of these claims are completely false, and others are looking at the wrong thing. For example, it's true that bad sunburns can increase your risk of skin cancer, but one study suggests the cause of these sunburns is likely a high intake of refined sugars and omega-6 fatty acids.[2] Another study reports that "Our results support the value of a systemic approach to identify specific sugars, and related cellular changes, that contribute to melanoma."[3] You need the vitamin D produced by exposure to sunlight for making cholesterol sulfates, and healthy vitamin D levels are important for a huge range of health benefits. You just need to change your diet so that you no longer are susceptible to severe sunburns.

This is just one example—the list goes on and on. There are many layers of this onion to peel back before we can understand the root cause of disease and what is truly harmful to us. However, let's start by examining how we got to where we are today.

HEALTHCARE AND PRESCRIPTIONS

Several components have contributed to the current state of healthcare in America. Some of these factors are political, some are systemic, and some are malicious manipulation of public opinion for the purpose of catering to corporate interests. Each of these components has led us to a healthcare environment in which a doctor is much more likely to write a prescription than to ask, "What are you eating?" Going into detail about each of these components could take up an entire book in itself, so we'll just touch on them here and provide references for further reading in case you're interested in the specifics.

The healthcare industry seems to believe that most of what ails us today—including cancer, obesity, metabolic syndrome, coronary artery disease, high cholesterol, Alzheimer's disease, dementia, ADHD, anxiety, and depression—is a result of genetic defects that are unavoidable. Although there are genetic components that can enhance your susceptibility to a particular disease or health issue, your genetic makeup doesn't doom you to one particular fate. Instead, your genetic makeup only increases the likelihood that you might develop a disease *if you give your body the wrong inputs.*

The healthcare industry looks at many diseases and other health conditions as being genetic, so they develop medications to treat the symptoms rather than going after the disease itself by suggesting that we change our foods. Because there is a profit motive behind the "solution"—prescription drugs—there is a strong motive to keep pushing that solution. We have found ourselves in this position for several reasons. Here are just a few:

- Scientific studies sometimes use flawed methods. For example, correlation does not equal causation (that is, just because two things are correlated doesn't mean that one caused the other).
- The industry's standard of care guidelines make them slow to change.
- Corporate lobbying influences government regulations.

TIP

I finally decided to become an advocate for health when I took our dog, Teva, to the vet because she was losing patches of hair. The first question the vet asked was, "What are you feeding her?" What a good question! Interestingly, that same week, I had to see my family physician for severe irritable bowel syndrome and acid reflux. My doctor tossed me some medication and sent me on my way.

You know what? My doctors have never asked me about what I am eating. Instead of following my doctor's advice to medicate myself to clear up the irritable bowel syndrome and acid reflux, I took the vet's advice and changed my diet (as well as my dog's). Soon enough, I was healed of my ailments, no drugs needed. Let food be thy medicine.

In the coming sections, we take a look at the corporate manipulation that has had a huge impact on nutritional guidance over the last fifty-plus years.

FLAWED DIETARY GUIDELINES

The dietary guidelines that have long been regarded as the undisputed truth come with the misconception that the health problems plaguing us today cannot be prevented. In the late 1970s, the U.S. Department of Agriculture (USDA) produced guidelines that emphasized keeping fat intake low while promoting consumption of more carbohydrates and lots of whole grains as ideal nutrition for longevity. They looked something like this:

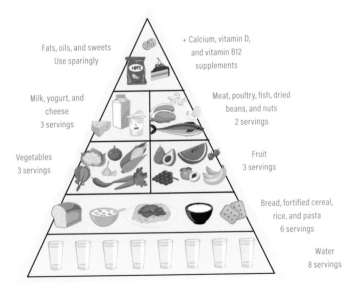

Ancel Keys was a researcher who famously hypothesized in the 1970s that diets high in saturated fat raise cholesterol, which leads to higher rates of coronary artery disease. His findings led to the development of the USDA guidelines. However, there are mountains of evidence today that show this hypothesis is false. When creating his report, Keys had reliable data that didn't align with his hypothesis, and we now know that he left out that data to better fit his agenda. In other words, bad science played a big part in the recommendation to eat low fat and lots of whole grains. Even more interesting is that corporate influence led to much of those recommendations.

Many political and corporate influences were in play, and it would take a whole book to outline them. Science writer Gary Taubes does just that in his books *The Case Against Sugar* and *Why We Get Fat*.[4,5] He explains in detail how corporate and political interests influenced what we've been told is the best way to eat. As a result, the food pyramid got just about everything wrong. In *The Case Against Sugar*, Taubes makes a strong case for how the sugar industry purposely drove the narrative away from sugar and toward saturated fat. In fact, we now have documents revealing that the sugar lobby paid large sums of money to fund studies in the 1970s with the objective of supporting claims that saturated fat leads to coronary artery disease.

A CBC News story written by Kelly Crowe reports on the efforts of a dentist named Cristin Couzens to uncover proof that the sugar industry had manipulated public opinion. Couzens found that for years the sugar industry had used tactics that mimicked those used by the tobacco industry. The sugar industry knew that their products were causing health issues and covered it up.[6]

"It's a little bit shocking to me that an industry would be rewarded for manipulating scientific evidence," Couzens said. "At the time the award was given in 1976, there was a controversy. Many people thought sugar was harmful, the sugar industry wanted to turn public opinion toward thinking sugar was safe so they forged public opinion on how the public viewed the effects of sugar."

A 2016 article written by Camila Domonoske and published by NPR discusses this deliberate action by the sugar industry.[7] It cites a study titled "Sugar Industry and Coronary Heart Disease

Research: A Historical Analysis of Internal Industry Documents," which states, "Our findings suggest the industry sponsored a research program in the 1960s and 1970s that successfully cast doubt about the hazards of sucrose while promoting fat as the dietary culprit in CHD [coronary heart disease]."[8]

A 2016 *New York Times* article by Anahad O'Connor describes this same study. "I think it's appalling," Marion Nestle, New York University professor of nutrition, food studies, and public health, says in the article. "You just never see examples that are this blatant."[9]

Domonoske's article also cites Nestle's commentary in the same issue of *JAMA Internal Medicine* in which the study was published:

> Is it really true that food companies deliberately set out to manipulate research in their favor? Yes, it is, and the practice continues. In 2015, the *New York Times* obtained emails revealing Coca-Cola's cozy relationships with sponsored researchers who were conducting studies aimed at minimizing the effects of sugary drinks on obesity. Even more recently, the Associated Press obtained emails showing how a candy trade association funded and influenced studies to show that children who eat sweets have healthier body weights than those who do not.

In a 2013 *National Geographic* article, Rich Cohen writes:

> "It seems like every time I study an illness and trace a path to the first cause, I find my way back to sugar." Richard Johnson, a nephrologist at the University of Colorado Denver, was talking to me in his office in Aurora, Colorado, the Rockies crowding the horizon. He's a big man with eyes that sparkle when he talks. "Why is it that one-third of adults [worldwide] have high blood pressure, when in 1900 only five percent had high blood pressure?" he asked. "Why did 153 million people have diabetes in 1980, and now we're up to 347 million? Why are more and more Americans obese? Sugar, we believe, is one of the culprits, if not the major culprit."[10]

Based on this evidence, we can conclude that much of the connection between saturated fat and coronary artery disease was forged by the sugar industry, which funded studies to support this claim with the motive of taking the spotlight off the real cause—sugar. And, as described in Domonoske's article, the manipulation is still going on today, which is tragic. The sugar industry knew that its products were harming people way back in the 1960s, yet it deliberately funded research to shift attention away from sugar so that it could sell more of those products that hurt people!

Before the manipulation of these facts in the 1960s and 1970s, it was common knowledge that sugar was harmful. The results of this manipulation are clear: Sugar-related illnesses and chronic diseases have skyrocketed while sugar industry profits have soared! The fear of fat led to the low-fat or fat-free product trend that dominated the 1980s and 1990s. What happens when you take out the fat? You need to replace it with sugar so your food still tastes good. Most prepackaged foods contain sugar. The following figure shows how sugar consumption in the U.S. has skyrocketed since the 1820s, according to a report from the Department of Commerce and the USDA.

U.S. SUGAR CONSUMPTION, 1822–2005

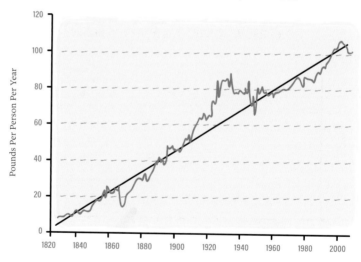

Source: United States Department of Commerce and USDA report

These sugar industry–funded studies falsely put the spotlight on saturated fat and cholesterol. The primary result was a vilification of saturated fat and cholesterol as the bad guys, which benefited the sugar industry because when you remove fat from foods, you have to replace it with sugar to make it more palatable.

This increased the added sugars in foods. A secondary result of this manipulation was that companies started to look for oils that were low in saturated fats, which led them to develop oils high in omega-6 fats, like vegetable and seed oils. Unfortunately, these oils are easily oxidized and cause inflammation in the body; a balance of omega-6 and omega-3 fats is important for keeping inflammation down. This increase in omega-6 oils might be just as damaging as the increase in sugar intake. As we discuss in the next chapter, inflammation is one of the main sources of many common diseases.

The following figure shows what has happened in the fifty years since the guidelines to avoid saturated fats and cholesterol were put into place; the result was a drastic reduction in butter and lard consumption and skyrocketing consumption of the purportedly "healthy" vegetable and seed oils that were recommended as replacements. These "heart-healthy" fats—such as canola oil, soybean oil, margarine, and vegetable shortening—were pumped into the food supply in alarming quantities. The figure also shows the alarming increases in processed foods, whereas consumption of foods like butter and lard decreased dramatically.

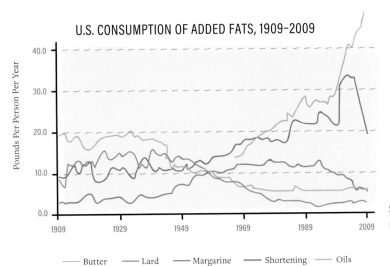

U.S. CONSUMPTION OF ADDED FATS, 1909–2009

Source: www.youtube.com/watch?v=HC200olgG_Y

In 1909, the most commonly used fat was butter; lard came in second. As you can see, starting in the 1950s, both butter and lard saw huge drops in consumption. The 1960s and 1970s saw the introduction of vegetable and seed oils, particularly soybean oil. By

NEGATIVE INFLUENCES ON NUTRITION

The influence by the sugar companies was just one of many factors that led to the disastrous state of health in our country. Other influences included the grain lobby's promotion of healthy whole grains and flawed study conclusions that showed that meat causes cancer.

2009, seed oils were by far the most commonly used fats, followed by vegetable shortening; butter and lard had moved to the bottom of the list.

Today, Americans have an average omega-3 to omega-6 ratio of 1:14 to 1:25. That means they get 14 to 25 times as much omega-6 as omega-3. A ratio closer to 1:1 is ideal for keeping inflammation low.

The healthcare industry just followed the guidance given to them by the American Medical Association and the FDA, which was flawed and heavily influenced by political and corporate interests. For decades, doctors and other healthcare providers recommended vegetable oils, low-fat diets, and "healthy" whole grains. When medical professionals recommended this "healthier" way of eating to their patients, many of those patients got sicker. Instead of blaming their recommendations, doctors instead blamed the patients and assumed that the patients weren't following the guidelines or that the patients were genetically damaged (in other words, bad genes made them gain weight). These assumptions led to the idea that medicines that cover the symptoms were the only course of action available.

We believe this is a big part of why our society pushes pills to solve problems. Many doctors believe "healthy nutrition" isn't working, so they prescribe a medicine to mask symptoms. However, here is the thing about prescriptions: They almost never address the root cause of the problem. Remember Craig's note from the beginning of the chapter? You have to get to the source—the input—of the problem and fix it so that the output is correct. If you continue giving your body bad inputs that lead to disease and symptoms, your doctor will attempt to mask those symptoms with a pill. If you don't address the root cause of the issue, you could end up taking that medication for the rest of your life. Of course, taking medicines for the rest of your life is good for the pharmaceutical companies' bottom lines, but it's not always good for your health.

The board is stacked against doctors today because they are taught flawed nutritional information. When doctors recommend a "healthy" (low-fat, high-carb) diet to patients, many see their patients' conditions worsen. Pharmaceutical companies lobby doctors with claims that their medications are cures when often they are just masking the symptoms.

Also, doctors must follow the "standard of care," which dictates that they follow a guideline for every patient with a given condition. For example, if a patient has a higher risk of coronary artery disease, the standard of care dictates that the doctor prescribe a statin medication to lower cholesterol. If the doctor goes against this standard of care, he or she could open himself or herself up to a lawsuit for not giving the "agreed upon best care for this condition." We know doctors who prescribe statins even though they no longer believe in their use. However, those doctors must follow the standard of care, or they could get in trouble. Think about the time limitations put on doctors to get people in and out the door as quickly as possible; when you do, it becomes obvious why the predominant solution is to write a prescription and move on. Doctors just don't have time to take action and fix the inputs (diet, lifestyle, and environment) that are the real cause of their patients' problems, which means physicians often simply write a prescription and move on to the next patient.

These issues have left us with ever-rising rates of obesity and chronic disease. Let's take a look at one of the most important inputs that cause these issues: diet. We'll start by looking at what the excess carbohydrates and empty calories in processed foods are doing to our bodies.

OVERCONSUMPTION OF CARBOHYDRATES

Here are just some of the things that result from eating too many refined carbohydrates:

- **Fatigue**: The most common feature of insulin resistance is that it causes exhaustion. Sometimes it's confined to just mornings or afternoons, but sometimes it's an all-day fatigue.
- **Brain fog:** Insulin resistance is often mental. The most evident symptom is an inability to concentrate. Poor memory and failing or poor grades in school are often a side effect of insulin resistance. Are you sending your kids off to school with a bowl of cereal and skim milk? If so, that's not a good idea.
- **Low blood sugar:** Feeling jittery and moody is common in insulin resistance; once you eat, you feel immediate relief.

Dizziness and a craving for sweets are also caused by low blood sugar.

- **Intestinal bloating**: Most intestinal gas is produced from too many carbohydrates. People with insulin resistance who eat carbohydrates suffer from gas—lots of it. Antacids or other remedies for symptomatic relief are not very successful in dealing with the problem.

- **Tired after meals**: The main side effect of consuming meals that contain more than 20 to 30 percent carbohydrates is being sleepy. Your meals are more than 20 to 30 percent carbs if they are pasta-based or include bread, potatoes, and a sweet dessert.

- **Increased fat storage and weight**: The most evident symptom in men is a large abdomen; in women, fat is stored on the hips and thighs.

- **Increased triglycerides**: Even people who aren't overweight can have excess fat in their arteries because of insulin resistance (see Chapter 3).

- **Increased blood pressure**: Doctors now recognize that most people with hypertension have too much insulin and are insulin resistant. There is often a direct relationship between insulin level and blood pressure. As insulin levels increase, so does blood pressure.

- **Depression**: Carbohydrates are a natural "downer," which depress the brain. Depressed people often also suffer from insulin resistance. Carbohydrates change the brain chemistry, producing a depressed or "tired" feeling. On the flip side, protein is a brain stimulant, which picks you up mentally.

- **Addiction**: Insulin resistance is also prevalent in people addicted to alcohol, caffeine, cigarettes, or other drugs. Often, the alcohol addiction is secondary to insulin resistance. The true addiction—sugar—was never kicked.

Many of our clients come to us after trying Weight Watchers. They find that it worked for a while, but now they've reached a weight plateau and can't lose more weight. Counting points isn't helpful for your biochemistry. Saving up all your points for a milkshake isn't going to enhance your physique. Even if you eat only 800 calories a day, those calories shouldn't come from trans fat and sugar! We don't understand the science behind giving 5 cups of plain popcorn only one point when that 5 cups of popcorn becomes more than 9 teaspoons of sugar in your blood. (Every 4 grams of carbohydrate becomes 1 teaspoon of sugar in the blood.) That sugar increases insulin—the fat-storing hormone—and kicks in other hormones that change your biochemistry, which causes more cravings for carbohydrates.

We all know that sugar is bad, but many people mistakenly believe complex carbohydrates are healthy and that they need to eat them in abundance. However, what if we told you that complex carbohydrates are just glucose molecules strung in long chains? The digestive track breaks them down into glucose (sugar), which means a sugary diet and a starchy diet are pretty much identical. When we say "sugar," we are also referring to starch.

Sugar is very gratifying. That first bite of heaven can calm us down and give us energy at the same time. It's like magic, and it has the power to flip your mood 180 degrees. That's the upside of sweets. The downside is that the more you eat, the more you want. Excess sugar causes a hormonal imbalance, which leads to carbohydrate cravings and weight gain, turning your body into a fat-making, fat-storing machine. However, we have good news for you. You are in charge, you can get off the fast track to diabetes, and you can do it naturally.

Overconsumption of fat-free foods and a sedentary life can lead to increased fat storage. When this fat storage gets too high (as described in Chapter 3) and adipose tissue (fat-storage sites) gets inflamed (hypertrophic, or overstuffed with fat), insulin resistance starts. Your body's primary way of getting rid of sugar is to burn it with exercise. The sugar your body can't burn is stored as glycogen, and when your glycogen reserves are full, the remaining sugar is stored as fat. Also, insulin prevents your body from burning fat. When you eat sugar, your body will burn the sugar rather than the stored fat. To learn more, see "Oxidative Priority" in Chapter 3.

Sugars are the simplest form of carbohydrate. Sugars come in natural forms, such as lactose (milk sugar) and fructose (fruit sugar), and in refined forms, such as sucrose (table sugar). All starchy foods (such as potatoes) and sweet foods (such as fresh fruit) raise blood sugar quickly. Sugar is immediately absorbed into your bloodstream, which causes insulin production to increase. Insulin clears sugar and fat from the blood; those sugars are then stored in your body tissues for future use, and all the fat is stored in fat cells, which results in weight gain.

No matter where the carbohydrates come from, four grams of carbohydrates equal one teaspoon of sugar. Let us say that again: Four grams of carbohydrates equal one teaspoon of sugar. The average American now gets more 300 grams of carbohydrates a day! This added sugar is mostly in the form of refined white sugar, which is high in calories and devoid of nutrients. Also, many prepackaged food contain hidden sugar. For instance, many varieties of bread contain refined sugar. Chocolate cake and other sweet delights can contain as much as 25 teaspoons of refined sugar—and that's not including the refined flour that is converted to sugar in your bloodstream! Even some salts contain maltodextrin, which is higher on the glycemic index (an index of how quickly a food raises blood sugar) than sugar!

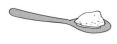

White sugar isn't the only danger; powdered sugar, honey, and maple syrup are also sources of refined sugar. Eating too much sugar is part of an addictive cycle. Sugar is quickly digested and burned, which causes peaks and valleys in your energy level and leaves you craving more sugar. When you eat too much sugar, your blood sugar spikes, which is followed by a drop in your blood sugar that makes you hungrier.

It is a dangerous situation when uninformed medical professionals recommend a high-complex-carbohydrate, low-saturated-fat diet. For all practical purposes, a high-complex-carbohydrate diet is nothing more than a high-blood-sugar diet.

TIP

Growing up, we had one TV that got only three channels. We only watched television in the evenings, and we watched what my parents wanted to watch. My mother loved *Little House on the Prairie.* I remember Laura Ingalls Wilder, the young girl portrayed in the show, getting one piece of candy each year at Christmas. The story takes place in the 1870s and 1880s. From an evolutionary perspective, that's not very long ago. Think about how much candy kids eat now. It is rare for them to go even one day without candy! I even had a client whose twelve-year-old son had type 1 diabetes, and when he scored 100 percent on his math test, the teacher gave him a jumbo-sized bag of candy!

Eggs for Breakfast?! But What About My Cholesterol Levels?

The most common misperception about cholesterol is that there's something unhealthy about it. Cholesterol is one of the body's repair substances, and its elevated presence in your system tells you that your body is trying to heal something. Often, that something is inflammation, which is the true source of the problem. Most Americans consume 200 to 300 milligrams of cholesterol a day, but your body needs around 1,000 milligrams a day, so your body produces the rest of the needed cholesterol in the liver, no matter what. Your body makes extra cholesterol because cholesterol is essential for hormone function, particularly the hormones your body needs during stressful times. When people use statin drugs to reduce their cholesterol—instead of focusing on eliminating the foods that cause the inflammation (processed foods)—it causes a wide range of side effects, including muscle fatigue, lowering of CoQ10 (an important vitamin for heart health), increased risk of diabetes, and much more. So give your liver a break and add some extra eggs!

Insulin is secreted in response to elevated blood sugar levels, such as those that occur after a meal. Insulin tries to push that sugar into storage. The body converts the sugar into glycogen to be stored in muscle and in the liver. Glycogen is the body's fuel of choice for high-intensity aerobic activity because it is readily available and because it is quickly converted to ATP (adenosine triphosphate), our bodies' energy units.

Insulin works to help your body preserve energy from food, and it does so in three ways:

- First, insulin tells your body to eat. When you eat sugar, your body rewards you with feelings of extreme gratification.

- Second, insulin escorts the energy from these foods to wherever your body needs it. Insulin tells the liver to turn any extra energy (once glycogen is full) into blood fat called triglycerides, which are stored in the fat cells.

- Lastly, insulin orders the body to keep the food energy locked inside the fat cells where it is stored rather than burning it for energy. In reality, your body must process carbs first—thanks to oxidative priority—so if you eat excess carbs, much of the fat is just stored while your body burns the carbs. The more sugar you eat, the more you crave it. If you start your day with cereal and skim milk, it is going to be hard to walk by the candy jar in your office at 2 p.m.

Check out these breakfast comparisons:

Option 1: 1 cup SMART START Cereal with 1 cup skim milk and a banana

472 calories, 105 grams carbs, 4 grams fiber = 25.25 teaspoons of sugar in the blood (if you didn't add any sugar!)

Option 2: 2 eggs with 2 cups of chopped mushrooms, peppers, and onions

190 calories, 9 grams carbs, 3 grams fiber = 1.5 teaspoons of sugar in the blood (This option will likely keep you full longer.)

SUGAR ACCELERATES AGING

In the past, access to concentrated forms of sugar was quite limited, so our bodies were not accustomed to dealing with it. Our bodies are placed under significant strain when they must process the large amounts of sugar that many people consume today. Excess sugar lingers in the blood and causes trouble by attaching to protein molecules via a process called glycation, where glycogen components are added to a protein. This results in the development of advanced glycation end-products (AGEs), which cause cellular aging in several ways:

- AGEs slow the body's repair mechanism. Although the effects are mostly internal, aging skin is a prime external sign. When excess blood sugar is causing AGEs to form, the skin loses its natural repair abilities. Sugar molecules clog up the collagen in your skin; reducing access to collagen means your skin is less elastic, wrinkles more quickly, and can't heal as quickly if it's damaged.

- AGEs age the body by spawning oxidative stress. The damage, called oxidation, causes inflammation. Eating poorly is like hitting the fast-forward button on aging because this chronic inflammation is the stem of most modern diseases.

- AGEs can cause cataracts.

- Even more troubling are new findings that show overconsumption of sugar (and development of AGEs) is linked to increased arterial plaque in people with heart disease, as well as in the brains of those with Alzheimer's disease and Parkinson's disease.

Few people can resist the taste of sweet foods. Food companies are well aware of this, so they add sugar to their products to get us hooked on their brands. Major sources of sugar include candy, cake, cookies, and fruit drinks, but sugar is hidden in a lot of so-called healthy foods, too. For example, some purportedly healthy frozen dinners can have as much sugar as three candy bars! And some fat-free yogurt contains more sugar per serving than a candy bar. You have to be a detective and root out the added sugars in your food.

PROBLEMS CAUSED BY TOO MUCH SUGAR

Excess sugar causes a variety of problems:

- **High blood pressure:** Insulin assists in the storage of excess energy as well as magnesium. However, if your cells become resistant to insulin, you can't store magnesium, which means you lose magnesium via urination. Also, intracellular magnesium relaxes muscles. When you can't store magnesium because the cell is resistant, you lose magnesium, and your blood vessels constrict, which leads to increased blood pressure.

- **Sodium retention and congestive heart failure:** High insulin also causes the retention of sodium, which leads to fluid retention; fluid retention causes high blood pressure and congestive heart failure.

- **Increased homocysteine:** A recent study showed that overweight children with high insulin levels are also likely to have high levels of homocysteine, a substance that appears to raise the risk of heart disease, stroke, and congenital problems.[11]

- **Osteoporosis:** Insulin is a master hormone that controls many anabolic hormones (hormones that stimulate growth), such as growth hormone, testosterone, and progesterone. Insulin resistance reduces the anabolic process. Anabolic hormones drive the formation of bone, so when these hormones are reduced, the building of bone is reduced, too. Also, when your body is always in sugar-burning mode, it needs a constant supply of glucose in the blood. But overnight everyone fasts for ten hours or more. So sugar-burners are more likely to begin using protein to convert to glucose (gluconeogenesis) to supply glucose. The sheath or covering of our bones is primarily made of proteins. Over time, this results in cannibalizing the bones' protein sheath, resulting in osteoporosis.

- **Increased cancer risk:** Insulin increases cellular reproduction, which increases your risk of cancer. One study has shown that increased insulin levels are one of the strongest correlations to breast and colon cancers.[12] Other research is showing that cancer thrives on glucose (called the Warburg effect) but isn't good at metabolizing fats.[13, 14]

FRUCTOSE AND METABOLISM

Have you looked at the ingredients in your barbecue sauce? The first ingredient is usually corn syrup—not tomatoes! Even if you make your own barbecue sauce using ketchup as the base, ketchup is still very high in sugar.

 You might be thinking, "Well, I don't buy the ketchup that contains high-fructose corn syrup. I get the organic agave-sweetened brands at health-food stores." But that alternative is no better. In fact, it might be even worse because agave is almost all fructose.

Like many sweeteners, agave syrup is marketed as being "low-glycemic," which is true; however, agave syrup is "low-glycemic" because of its shockingly high concentration of fructose. Following are the makeup of sugars in some common sweeteners:

- Agave syrup is 90 percent fructose and 10 percent glucose.
- High-fructose corn syrup ranges from 55 to 65 percent fructose.
- Honey is about 55 percent fructose.
- Sugar (that is, standard table sugar) is 50 percent fructose and 50 percent glucose.

Fructose is harmful for many reasons, including the following:

- **Only the liver can process fructose.** Fructose can be metabolized only by the liver; glucose, on the other hand, can be metabolized by every cell in the body. Fructose bypasses the enzyme phosphofructokinase, which is the rate-limiting enzyme for glucose metabolism. The liver converts this fructose to glucose or fat, which, unfortunately, remains in the liver and can lead to fatty liver disease. Overconsumption of fructose is why we see so many children with fatty liver disease. They aren't drinking alcohol; they are drinking sodas and juices and, in general, consuming too much fructose!

- **Increased uric acid leads to higher blood pressure and gout.** Fructose is high in uric acid, which increases blood pressure and causes gout.

- **Fructose accelerates oxidative damage and increases aging.** Fructose changes the collagen of your skin, making it prone to wrinkles.

- **Consumption of large amounts of fructose leads to mineral loss.** A high intake of fructose leads to loss of minerals—including iron, calcium, magnesium, and zinc—which in turn can lead to low bone density (osteoporosis). High fructose levels also interfere with copper metabolism, which prevents the formation of collagen and elastin, the connective tissues that hold our bodies together. A deficiency in copper can also lead to infertility, bone loss, anemia, defects of the arteries, infertility, high cholesterol, heart attacks, and an inability to control blood sugar.

- **Eating fructose doesn't trigger your brain to send a "stop eating" signal.** Fructose does not affect the production of ghrelin, the hunger hormone. Fructose also interferes with the brain's communication with leptin, which is the hormone that tells you to stop eating. You can become leptin resistant! (See Chapter 5 to learn more.)

So don't swap out sugar for more fructose. This will lower the insulin response but won't make you healthier—and may even make you sicker. Eliminating all sugars is the best course of action for lowering your carbohydrate intake, getting insulin-signaling under control, and healing your body.

In this book, we look at the basic biology of the human body. We show you how it processes different fuel sources and how it controls the flow in and out of your fat cells. We also explain how the disruption in the body's signaling (insulin) causes metabolic disease to start in the fat cells (adipose tissues) and look at the true root causes of disease and how changing the inputs (these root causes) can reverse many of the diseases that plague us today.

FOOD MARKETING AND NUTRITION

Food companies often employ marketing geniuses who come up with slogans such as "Heart Smart." However, food manufacturers often add way too many cheap fillers, like high-fructose corn syrup, to their products to make them more palatable so that you eat more. A product labeled as "Heart Smart" might contain 10 grams of sugar in one tiny serving, and sugar isn't "heart smart." Sugar causes inflammation, which is the real cause of heart disease.

chapter 2

The Disease Tree

Many common diseases are preventable or reversible. The things we put into our bodies—the inputs—are the root cause of these diseases. When we put the wrong things into our bodies, our bodies begin to fail, resulting in disease.

In this chapter, we first look at the things that cause a disruption in insulin signaling. Then we look at what you can do to reverse this disruption.

The following disease tree shows the process by which some common diseases originate:

- The roots represent the root causes that make our bodies break down.
- The tree trunk represents insulin and other hormone signaling. Disruption of insulin signaling is a major player in metabolic failures and disease progression.
- The leaves represent the end results: the disease.

FINDING THE ROOT CAUSES OF DISEASE

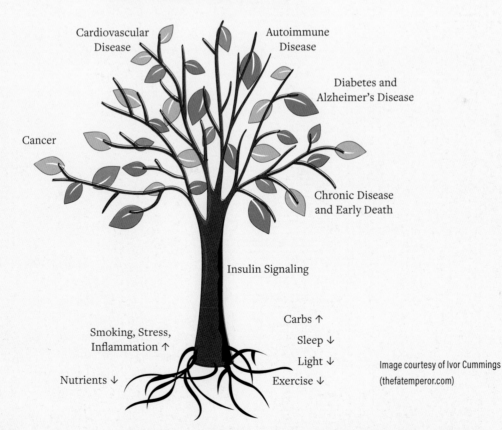

Cardiovascular Disease

Autoimmune Disease

Diabetes and Alzheimer's Disease

Cancer

Chronic Disease and Early Death

Insulin Signaling

Smoking, Stress, Inflammation ↑

Carbs ↑

Sleep ↓

Light ↓

Nutrients ↓

Exercise ↓

Image courtesy of Ivor Cummings (thefatemperor.com)

Many inputs can contribute to the proliferation of disease, some more so than others. Let's break down some of the key issues:

- **Smoking:** We all know smoking is deadly. We don't have much to say here except if you smoke, quit.

- **Stress:** Stress is a contributing factor in many diseases. It raises cortisol and can increase inflammation in the body. Reducing stress can lower inflammation, improve immune response, and reduce the risk of many common diseases.

- **Inflammation:** Chronic inflammation is a major cause of most diseases. As we discuss in Chapter 1, the nutritional advice we have been given over the last fifty years has led many people to living in a chronic state of inflammation. Overconsumption of sugar and omega-6 oils leads to inflammation, which leads to diseases such as coronary artery disease. Reducing inflammation is critical to improving your health.

- **Low nutrient density:** When you eat foods with low nutrient density, your body isn't getting the nutrients it needs. Your body then continues sending hunger signals, which leads to overeating. Nutrient-dense foods trigger satiety and keep you full longer while giving your body all the nutrients it needs to keep your cells healthy.

- **Excess carbohydrates:** See Chapters 1 and 3 to learn more about how excess carbohydrate intake is a major contributor to metabolic diseases.

- **Sleep:** Getting enough sleep is another important contributor to health. Studies have shown that just going from eight hours of sleep to four hours of sleep doubled the insulin resistance of U.S. army personnel.[1] Failure to get enough sleep also leads your body to send hunger signals, which cause you to overeat.

- **Exercise:** Exercise is also very important, but not in the way you might think. The average American walks only a mile or so a day (spread out throughout the day during normal tasks). We are not telling you to run on a treadmill; however, the more activity you can get, the better. Little movements—such as walking to the mailbox, parking at the back of the lot at the grocery store, and using the stairs instead of taking the elevator or escalator—add up. The more you move throughout the day, the more energy from your fat stores is consumed, making it less likely that fat cells become inflamed (more on that in the next section). Also, exercise is one of the best ways to increase autophagy, which is your body's process for cleaning up old or failing cells. Autophagy breaks down old and failing cells and makes new, healthier cells (think of this as a cellular reversing of aging). Exercise also builds new mitochondria, the energy-burning centers in our cells.

- **Light:** Another component of healthfulness is light. Humans evolved as a species bathed in light. We are not used to climate-controlled buildings devoid of natural light. Much research shows that lack of sunlight exposure can cause many issues.

INFLAMED ADIPOSE TISSUE CAUSES INSULIN RESISTANCE

The constant flow of fat in and out of our fat cells is called *fat flux* (see Chapter 3). Fat flux is a normal process in which fat enters the fat cells when the blood contains excess fat that isn't burned as fuel. (Excess carbohydrates that have been converted to fat also enter the fat cells, to a lesser extent.) Fat flux includes both dietary fat and excess fat that has been removed from the fat cells through a process called *lipolysis*. It is a continual process in which fat is always entering our cells; when lipolysis is enabled, fat also moves out of the fat cells to be used to fuel our bodies.

Our fat cells can hold only so many fat molecules (triglycerides or stored fat composed of three free fatty acids linked together by a glycerol molecule). When a fat cell is overstuffed with fat molecules, it becomes inflamed.[2] The fat cell can't hold any more fat molecules and becomes insulin resistant (meaning that it won't allow any more fat in). If too many of your fat cells become insulin resistant, your metabolism starts to fail, and a chain reaction occurs:

1. The fat levels in your blood (triglycerides) start to rise.
2. Your liver attempts to package the excess fat into triglycerides so that they can be stored in fat cells.

METABOLIC SYNDROME

Metabolic syndrome is a condition that increases the risk for a range of issues, including diabetes, stroke, heart disease, high blood pressure, high blood sugar, excess body fat, and high triglycerides. Essentially, metabolic syndrome is a precursor to type 2 diabetes.

3. When your fat cells won't allow any additional fat to enter, triglycerides continue to rise. Your body also starts putting out more insulin.

4. The lower levels of insulin don't drive down the levels of fat and carbohydrates, so the body outputs more insulin (the hormone that drives fuel into cells and storage) in an attempt to lower the levels of glucose, fat, and so on in the blood.

5. Because the fat cells aren't taking in fat, more fat accumulates in the liver and pancreas.

6. This process causes a metabolic breakdown—which is insulin resistance and metabolic syndrome—starting in your fat cells.

When you think about it, this chain of events makes perfect sense. The inflamed and overstuffed fat cells being the primary starting point for insulin resistance explains why some thin people have type 2 diabetes. Thin diabetics don't have a lot of fat cells, but the ones they do have are stuffed and inflamed. On the other hand, some people who are overweight don't have diabetes because they don't have a lot of inflamed fat cells (yet).

Modern science isn't clear on why some people have—or can make—more fat cells while others can't. One theory is that we don't make many new fat cells after a young age. When we are young, we can make more fat cells, but at some point, we don't make many more cells; instead, we just fill the ones we already have. Someone who was overweight as a child has more fat cells to fill and thus can gain more weight before the cells become inflamed.

However, we do know that when fat cells stop accepting fat and insulin rises, the liver pushes out more triglycerides so that they can be sent to your fat cells; the fat cells, however, aren't accepting the triglycerides, so the liver and pancreas accumulate more fat. At some point, your pancreas and beta cells (cells in the pancreas that produce insulin) just burn out and stop making insulin, and you become a type 2 diabetic.

To reverse insulin resistance and metabolic syndrome, you must shrink your fat cells and reverse the process, which means you need lipolysis to pull the fat from the fat stores and burn it as fuel. The ketogenic lifestyle can be a great tool for ramping up lipolysis and reversing insulin resistance.

WHAT ABOUT CHOLESTEROL?

Many doctors use cholesterol levels as a primary indicator of health. Let's look at why your cholesterol levels are pretty much meaningless.

First, let's consider what cholesterol is and what it does. As we discuss in more detail in Chapter 3, there are two primary fuel sources for the body:

- Glucose
- Free fatty acids (FFA) and, to a lesser extent, ketones made from FFA

Glucose can travel around the bloodstream on its own. However, neither cholesterol nor triglycerides can circulate in the blood without a carrier. Your body packages cholesterol and triglycerides in a carrier (think of a boat) called a low-density lipoprotein, or LDL. In general, the larger the LDL particle, the more triglyceride it contains.

As we've discussed, fat flux is a process in which the body pulls fat from fat stores. Leftover fat not burned by your muscles or other tissues is returned to the liver to be packaged into very-low-density lipoprotein (VLDL) particles; those VLDL particles are then sent back to the fat cells for storage. The amount of LDL (and total cholesterol) can be greatly influenced by the amount of fat in your diet. Your LDL levels will go down if you are keto-adapted because in that case fat is your primary fuel, and you are eating a lot of fat. When your diet consists of adequate fat, your LDL level drops because not as much fuel needs to be pulled from the fat cells. Alternatively, if you are in an energy deficit and eating fewer calories than your body needs, your LDL level goes up as your body pulls more fat from storage to use for fuel.

Dave Feldman is an engineer who has experimented with manipulating his cholesterol numbers via his diet. In his experiments, he eats a low-carb, moderate-protein diet and varies only the amount of fat he consumes. First he eats lower fat (1,000 total calories) and measures his cholesterol; then for three days he eats a great deal of fat (4,000 or more total calories) and measures his cholesterol again. Feldman has been able to take his small LDL-P (small LDL particle number)—which healthcare professionals consider to be the factor most indicative of coronary artery disease risk—from almost 1,000 (high risk) to below 90 (very low risk). He did this in just three days by doing the opposite of what you would think would be the healthy approach (based on conventional nutritional wisdom). When his LDL-P was 1,000, he was eating little fat and about 1,000 total calories. When his LDL-P was 90, he was eating upward of 350 grams of fat a day![3]

We could spend a whole chapter discussing the flawed correlation between cholesterol and coronary artery disease. Instead, let's look at a couple of highlights before we get into what you should really be looking at—a coronary artery calcium (CAC) test.

LDL cholesterol is the body's repair mechanism, and it facilitates fuel transportation. Coronary artery disease occurs when an LDL particle gets lodged in a lesion of the artery wall and releases its cholesterol to start repairing the lesion. The cholesterol develops into a plaque that seals up the lesion. However, over time, this plaque can block the artery and cause a heart attack. When the body produces this plaque, it's doing exactly what it should do; this process isn't flawed, and it's not a genetic mistake. If you had a hole in a wall of your house, what would you do? You would cover

STATINS

In the 1980s, my dad was prescribed a cholesterol medication—generically called a statin—as a preventive measure because he'd had one "high" cholesterol test. He took that statin for more than thirty years and suffered muscle soreness, joint pain, and other symptoms for most of that time. A couple of years ago, he finally decided to stop taking the statin. Then he had to go to the hospital for a minor stroke-like event. After a full year off the cholesterol medication, his total cholesterol was 180, which is in the desirable range, but the first thing the doctor advised my dad after the health incident was that he should go back on the statin.

I truly believe that we will someday look back at statins as pointless drugs that helped almost no one while they damaged many lives with increased diabetes rates and uncomfortable side effects. It breaks my heart that my dad had to spend thirty years of his life taking them.

the hole with spackle. That is exactly what your body is doing. If it didn't, the lesion could burst and kill you.

However, the lesion wasn't caused by the cholesterol. The cholesterol is like a firefighter coming to put out a fire; the firefighter didn't start the fire. Inflammation caused the lesion, and cholesterol patched it. The goal is preventing future fires (addressing the root cause of inflammation) rather than reducing the number of firefighters (cholesterol).

Cholesterol also performs many vital roles in the body. Following are some of the benefits of saturated fat and cholesterol.

THE BENEFITS OF SATURATED FAT

Saturated fat is not the cause of modern disease. On the contrary, it plays many vital roles in your body's chemistry:

- **It creates strong cell membranes.** Saturated fatty acids make up at least 50 percent of the cell membrane; they give cells stiffness and integrity.
- **It helps build strong bones.** Saturated fat plays a vital role in bone health. It is needed for calcium to be effectively incorporated into the skeletal structure.
- **It protects the liver against alcohol and other toxins.**
- **It improves the immune system.** Your white blood cells need adequate amounts of saturated fat to properly recognize and destroy foreign invaders like viruses, bacteria, and fungi.
- **It protects the digestive tract.** Saturated fat has antimicrobial properties that protect against harmful microorganisms in the digestive tract.

THE BENEFITS OF CHOLESTEROL

Our blood vessels become damaged due to irritation caused by free radicals or because they are structurally weak. When the blood vessels are damaged, the body's natural healing substance—cholesterol—steps in to repair the damage. Cholesterol is manufactured in your liver and cells. Like saturated fat, the cholesterol you make and consume plays many vital roles in your body:

- **It creates strong cell membranes.** Cholesterol, along with saturated fats, gives our cells required stiffness and stability.

When your diet contains an excess of polyunsaturated fats (vegetable oils or omega-6), the cell walls become weak. If the cell walls are weakened, cholesterol from the blood drives into the tissues to give them structural integrity. This process explains why serum cholesterol levels might go down temporarily when you replace saturated fats with polyunsaturated fats.

- **It improves serotonin levels.** Cholesterol is vital for the production and function of serotonin receptors in the brain. Serotonin is the body's "feel-good" chemical. Low cholesterol levels have been linked to depression and aggression.

- **It is a building block for critical hormones.** Cholesterol is a key building block for important hormones that help us deal with stress and protect us against cancer and heart disease. It is also important to our sex hormones: androgen, testosterone, estrogen, and progesterone.

- **It allows your body to utilize vitamin D.** Cholesterol is necessary for us to use vitamin D, which is an essential fat-soluble vitamin needed for healthy bones and nervous system, insulin production, reproduction and immune system function, proper growth, mineral metabolism, and muscle tone.

- **It creates bile.** Bile is made from the cholesterol we ingest and is vital for digestion and assimilation of fats in the diet.

- **It acts as an antioxidant.** Studies show that cholesterol is an antioxidant, which is why cholesterol levels tend to increase with age. As an antioxidant, cholesterol protects us against free-radical damage that can lead to heart disease and cancer.

- **It helps maintain intestinal health.** Cholesterol helps maintain the health of the intestinal wall. People on low-cholesterol vegetarian diets often develop leaky gut syndrome and other intestinal disorders.

Cholesterol is not the enemy it is made out to be. Let's look at some indicators that are far better than cholesterol at assessing your risk of coronary artery disease and other diseases.

WHAT MARKERS SHOULD YOU USE TO DETERMINE YOUR HEALTH?

If your cholesterol numbers don't really tell you anything, what markers do tell you the state of your health? There are several that are very useful.

CORONARY ARTERY CALCIUM SCORE (CAC)

By far the best predictor of coronary artery disease (CAD) is your coronary artery calcium (CAC) score. To get a CAC score, doctors image the arteries around the heart (the coronary arteries). Then they highlight the plaque in those arteries and give it a score based on the amount of plaque found. Scores range from zero to 1,000 or higher, with zero meaning little risk and a higher score meaning more plaque and higher risk. A calcium score is a direct measure of the disease, and it has a very high correlation to risk. The following figure shows the correlation of calcium score to CAD risk.[4]

CAC RISK

GROUP, CAC RISK CATEGORY	MODEL 1
All-cause mortality (*n* = 56)	
0	1.000
1–100	3.03 (0.62–14.92)
101–1,000	8.26 (1.86–36.68)
> 1,000	16.17 (3.64–71.75)
Cardiovascular disease endpoint (*n* = 127)	
0	1.000
1–100	1.92 (0.89–4.18)
101–1,000	2.23 (1.04–4.76)
> 1,000	7.51 (3.60–15.68)
Coronary heart disease endpoint (*n* = 67)	
0	1.000
1–100	1.42 (0.41–4.92)
101–1,000	3.13 (1.01–9.69)
> 1,000	9.97 (3.32–29.89)

As you can see, using a calcium score of zero as the reference, your risk for all causes of death with a calcium score of 1 to 100 is 300 percent higher than a score of zero. A calcium score of 101 to 1,000 means that your death risk is 826 percent higher; a score topping 1,000 means that your risk is 1,617 percent higher. Compare this to the statin companies' studies showing 3 percent or less correlation to risk with higher cholesterol levels, and you must ask yourself why you would even test your cholesterol levels.

The calcium score is the real predictor of coronary artery disease risk because it directly measures the plaque in your arteries—it doesn't just guess at the amount of plaque that might be there based on your cholesterol numbers. This test also points out the flaws associated with using cholesterol as a predictor of risk because people with cholesterol levels in the 400s might have a calcium score of zero, meaning that they have no plaque in their arteries and therefore little or no risk of CAD. However, people with very low cholesterol scores might have very high calcium scores and a very high risk of CAD.

If you want to know your real risk of CAD, get a calcium score. This test is usually pretty cheap (about $100) and can be done at most imaging centers and clinics.

- If your score is zero, great! Consider having a second test done in ten years or so.
- If your score is high, we recommend starting a well-formulated ketogenic diet right away to lower inflammation, as well as supplementing with the MK7 form of vitamin K2. Vitamin K2 regulates calcium metabolism and helps get calcium where it should be—in your bones—and prevents it from forming as plaque in your arteries.

KRAFT INSULIN TEST

Most physicians use a glucose tolerance test to check for diabetes. The problem with this test is that your metabolism must be pretty much broken before you will fail the test.

Dr. Joseph Kraft developed the Kraft Insulin Test, which measures insulin response instead of glucose response. This is a significant difference because the standard glucose tolerance test measures blood glucose over time after an oral dose of glucose.

You could show a normal return of blood glucose to baseline with a glucose test, but your body could be using a lot of insulin to force the glucose down, an early sign of insulin resistance. The Kraft Test measures insulin response after an oral glucose dose so you can see how much insulin is needed to bring down blood glucose. The following figure shows the different results you can get. Kraft found that there are four distinct profiles.

KRAFT PATTERNS: THE EARLIEST DIAGNOSIS OF DIABETES[5]

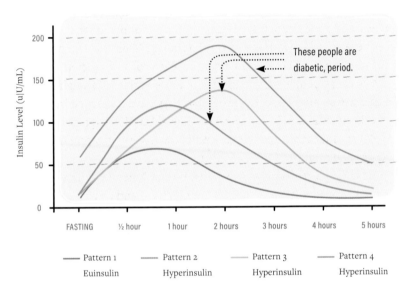

In the figure, Pattern 1, the lowest profile, is a normal insulin response; there is no sign of metabolic damage or diabetes. Patterns 2 and 3 show a person who needs more and more insulin to return to normal glucose levels. The body has to produce much more insulin to drive down blood glucose to normal levels. This is an early sign of insulin resistance. Pattern 4, the highest curve, is where a blood glucose test would finally fail. The body is producing massive amounts of insulin but still can't drive blood sugar levels down to a normal level.

The key here is that you won't fail a glucose tolerance test until you reach the highest curve, in which your body is putting out tons of insulin but still can't keep blood sugar down. Using a test like this can help identify the effects of insulin resistance much earlier than with a glucose test. The Kraft Test has been shown to reveal insulin resistance up to ten years before a glucose test is failed.

Many doctors will be able to help you get this test done, but if your doctor is resistant to ordering it or isn't familiar with it, you can get it done on your own for about $200. Meridianvalleylab.com even has a version that you can do at home.

A1C TEST

An A1c test estimates average blood glucose levels over a three-month period, which is a great indicator of how well you have managed your blood glucose and your overall health. The following figure shows that higher A1c levels mean an increased likelihood of cardiovascular disease or stroke. As you can see, those with A1c over 6.5 had more than five times the risk of cardiovascular disease and almost nine times the risk for stroke.

CORRELATION OF HEART DISEASE TO A1C LEVELS

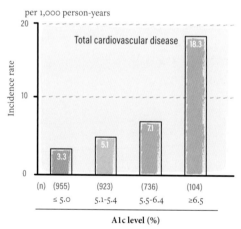

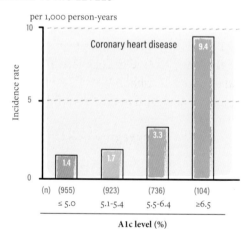

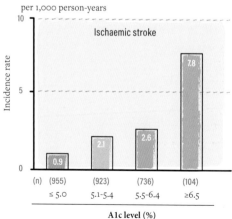

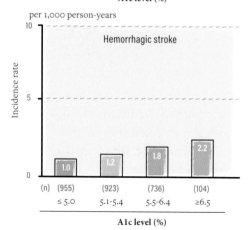

A1c also has a strong correlation to cancer. As shown in the graph below, those with A1c of 6.5 or higher had a 43 percent higher chance of getting cancer than those with A1c of 5.0 to 5.4.

HAZARD RATIO FOR CANCER RELATIVE TO A1C LEVELS

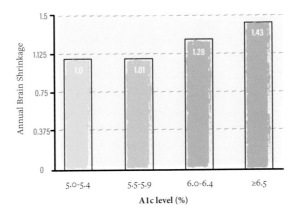

There is also a correlation between A1c and brain shrinkage as we age. This can lead to cognitive issues like Alzheimer's disease and dementia. Higher A1c levels are consistent with more brain shrinkage, as shown in the following figure.

BRAIN SHRINKAGE INCREASES WITH HIGHER A1C LEVELS[6]

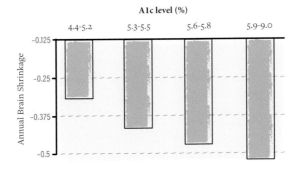

A1c can be an indicator of risk for many diseases, including metabolic syndrome and diabetes. An A1c level of 6.5 or higher is considered diabetic. However, the treatment target for people with diabetes is 7.0 or less.

As you can see, you want your A1c to be less than 5.3; ideally, you want it to be less than 5.0. Even type 1 diabetics following the ketogenic diet routinely see A1c levels below 5.0.

HIGHER TRIGLYCERIDE/HDL RATIOS AND HEART ATTACK RISK

Harvard Medical School has confirmed the importance of the triglyceride-to-HDL ratio. A higher TG/HDL ratio means that you are more likely to have a heart attack. In the 2004 study "Association of triglyceride-to-HDL cholesterol ratio with heart rate recovery," the researchers reported that participants in the highest quartile of the TG/HDL ratio were sixteen times more likely to have a heart attack than those in the lowest quartile![7]

TRIGLYCERIDE-TO-HDL RATIO

Triglyceride-to-HDL ratio (TG/HDL) is reported on the standard cholesterol panel that most doctors run as part of a regular checkup or yearly physical. A ratio of less than 2.0 means that you are doing well; ideally, you want to have this number be 1.0 or lower.

VITAMIN D LEVELS

Many Americans, especially those who live in northern climates, are deficient in vitamin D. Optimally, your vitamin D level should be at least 50 ng/ml. Low vitamin D levels have been associated with osteopenia and osteoporosis, many forms of cancer, heart disease, high blood pressure, multiple sclerosis, arthritis, depression, fibromyalgia, chronic pain, psoriasis, and much more.

Most people today slather on sunscreen the minute they go out into the sun. As we describe later in this chapter, some commonsense, healthy sun exposure can be very helpful for improving vitamin D levels. Vitamin D from the sun is the healthiest and most natural form you can get, and it comes with a lot of additional benefits.

REVERSING THE ROOT CAUSES

Let's look at how you can work on reversing the root causes of disease, shrink your adipose tissue, and restore your health.

SPENDING TOO MUCH TIME INDOORS CAN LEAD TO LOW VITAMIN D LEVELS

We brought our boys home from Ethiopia when they were one and two years old. Even though Ethiopia is on the equator, we had their vitamin D levels checked when we got them home, and both had very low levels of the vitamin. Their lower vitamin D levels were partly attributable to their darker skin, which makes getting enough vitamin D from sun exposure more difficult. However, we believe their low vitamin D levels were also caused by the fact that they spent a lot of time indoors at the orphanage and got only a little outdoor playtime.

STOP SMOKING

Stop. Just stop smoking.

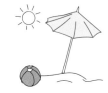

REDUCE STRESS

We lead busy lives that involve a lot of stressors, including work, kids, keeping the family and home running, long commutes, and so much more. Managing the stress of daily life has become increasingly important to maintaining good health.

There are many ways to manage stress levels. One of the best is to take a vacation! On average, the United States has one of the lowest vacation rates in the developed world. Many countries have mandatory vacations of six weeks or more. For example, Germany mandates a minimum of thirty-four days of vacation and holidays, whereas France and New Zealand both require at least thirty days.

Worse still is that many of us don't even take the meager amount of vacation time we have earned! In 2016, 54 percent of Americans didn't use all their vacation days, and more than one-third of those vacation days weren't paid out or rolled over—meaning they were just surrendered. We Americans work hard and are very productive. We need to take the time we have earned to recharge our batteries and reduce stress, even if our vacation is a "staycation" (a vacation at home).

Another way to reduce stress is to meditate or do yoga. Yoga is great for flexibility; it also allows you to spend time reflecting, calming yourself, and de-stressing.

Finally, set aside some time each day to unplug and commit to your family. Turn off your phone for a couple of hours and disconnect from work, email, and social media.

REDUCE INFLAMMATION AND LOWER CARBOHYDRATES

We lump inflammation and lowering carbohydrates together because they are directly related. Inflammation—including inflamed fat cells as well as the inflammation in arteries that leads to the formation of plaque—is behind most diseases. The root cause of nearly every major disease can be traced back to chronic inflammation.

A ketogenic lifestyle can help lower inflammation by reducing intake of sugar and carbohydrates and greatly reducing consumption of omega-6 fatty acids. We cover inflammation and lowering carbohydrate intake in more depth in Chapter 4.

INCREASE NUTRIENT DENSITY

Increasing the nutrient density of your diet can have many health benefits, including the following:

- Nutrient-dense foods increase satiety, which helps you avoid overeating.
- In general, nutrient-dense foods contain less sugar and carbohydrate, which helps reduce insulin needs and improves satiety.
- As we discuss in Chapter 8, some of the most nutrient-dense foods—animal proteins—contain no carbs.
- Eating nutrient-dense foods provides your body with the vitamins and minerals it needs, with fewer calories coming along for the ride. Most processed foods do the opposite, even though they are high in calories: Because they lack nutrients, eating them leaves you wanting more because your body isn't getting the nutrients it is looking for. Nutrient-dense foods give you the "I'm full" signal much more quickly, meaning that you consume fewer calories.

GET ENOUGH SLEEP

Not getting enough sleep can be very damaging, especially over the long term. Lose enough sleep and it can kill you! Our bodies do a bunch of beneficial things while we sleep, including producing human growth hormone (HGH).

Where to Find Nutrient-Dense Foods

Avoiding foods that are lacking in nutrients typically means staying away from the center aisles of the grocery store and sticking to the perimeter. Prepackaged foods are often devoid of nutrients but are high in calories. The outside walls of the store are where you will find nutrient-dense vegetables and animal proteins.

During deep sleep, our bodies produce HGH, which helps us do such things as heal from cuts, recover from workouts, and build new muscle. Stop consuming calories at least two hours before bedtime because eating too close to bedtime can interfere with the secretion of HGH and other hormones while you sleep. Eating an early dinner and then closing up the kitchen until morning is a great way to increase HGH (also known as the fat-burning hormone) as you snooze.

Like ocean waves, our hormones go up and down throughout the day. Insulin and HGH are antagonists, and because insulin is the stronger and more powerful of the two, it always wins. If you eat carbohydrates, insulin rises and therefore shunts the rise of HGH. The largest natural surge of HGH occurs thirty to seventy minutes after you fall asleep. However, if you just ate a bowl of ice cream or toast with peanut butter and honey (something Maria always did as a kid), you prevent that precious fat-burning hormone from helping you burn fat. By the time you wake up in the morning, you still have glycogen in your liver, and you haven't burned any fat at all.

Getting just five or six hours of sleep a night can cause issues, too. When you get an adequate amount of sleep, your body stimulates the production of leptin, the hormone that makes you feel full, and suppresses ghrelin, the hormone that makes you feel hungry. Also, there is evidence that our brains flush waste through the lymphatic system up to ten times faster during deep sleep than when we are awake.

So get some sleep! Try for eight to ten hours every night. Here are some tips to help you sleep better:

- **Keep your bedroom cool at night.** We keep ours at about 60°F. You can also try placing a cooling pad (we love our ChiliPad!) under your sheets to keep you cool.

- **Block out all sunlight.** Get blackout blinds to eliminate all light from the room, and cover up LED lights from electronic devices. (Better yet, banish them from the room entirely!)

- **Use a sound machine or fan.** White noise from a sound machine or a fan can help prevent you from being awakened by other sounds.

- **Wear blue-blocking sunglasses in the evening.** Your eyes have blue light receptors that connect to the suprachiasmatic nucleus (SCN) in your brain. When blue light is present, those receptors tell the SCN not to release melatonin, the hormone that makes you sleepy. When blue light isn't hitting your eyes, the SCN releases melatonin to make you feel drowsy and help you fall asleep. Today's artificially lit homes, along with smartphones, computers, tablets, and TVs, put out lots of blue light. Wearing blue light–blocking glasses can block this flood of blue light in the evening when you're ready for your body to be producing melatonin to make you sleepy. We recommend wearing them for three to four hours before you normally go to bed. You can purchase simple blue light–blocking safety glasses online for about $20. They are a good investment for better sleep!

EXERCISE DAILY

Exercise is the biggest stimulator of autophagy, which is the body's process for breaking down old and failing cells into their components and then building new, healthier cells from those parts. Fasting increases autophagy, although nothing increases it like strength training.[8] Strength training creates micro-tears in muscle tissue, and when this happens, your body turns up autophagy to help repair and rebuild those tissues by breaking down old tissue. In essence, exercise turns back the cellular aging clock.

Autophagy is one of the reasons strength training is so important. Maintaining lean muscle mass as we age is very important for vitality and strength. Strength training is good for people of any age.

GET SOME SUN

Over the last thirty to forty years, we have been told to avoid the sun at all costs and to slather on sunscreen whenever we are exposed to the sun's rays. As a result, sunscreen sales have skyrocketed. This increased sunscreen use must mean that the number of cases of melanoma has gone down, right? Not at all. In reality, rates of melanoma have skyrocketed as well, as shown in the following figure.

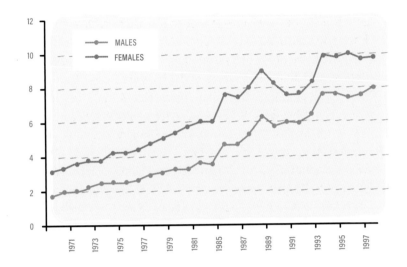

Melanoma rates have gone up more than 400 percent since the 1970s, which is the opposite of what you would expect if sunscreen was the answer to melanoma prevention.

A Swedish study evaluated sun exposure in relation to all causes of death, and the results actually showed an inverse relationship to sun exposure![9] The researchers learned that the less sun the participants got, the more likely they were to die. Another study showed that people living in Japan often get melanoma on the soles of their feet, which almost never are exposed to direct sunlight.[10] In 2000, yet another study showed that people who always use sunscreen have almost twice the rates of melanoma rates as those who never use it.[11]

Now, we aren't saying that there is zero correlation between sun exposure and skin cancer. Some types of skin cancer—the "cosmetic" cancers—do increase when you get the kinds of sunburns that make you blister. However, these "cosmetic" cancers are very treatable and have a death rate of about 0.5 percent, whereas melanomas have a death rate of about 50 percent (100 times higher!). Also, many other factors contribute to those higher melanoma death rates, including the chemicals in sunscreen and poor dietary choices, such as consuming excess omega-6 fatty acids and sugar.

Commonsense sun exposure can be very beneficial. Vitamin D deficiency is becoming a huge problem; it has been linked to increased risks for many conditions, including depression, dementia, heart disease, impaired immune function, high blood pressure, chronic pain, arthritis, metabolic syndrome, fibromyalgia, psoriasis, seventeen types of cancer, and even multiple sclerosis. You want your vitamin D levels to be 50 ng/ml or higher, but less than 100 ng/ml.

Some people say that we can replace sun exposure with vitamin D supplements. Yes, vitamin D supplements can be helpful seasonally for people who live in northern climates and can't get good sun exposure in the winter. However, most of these supplements contain only 2,000 or 5,000 IU of vitamin D, whereas just fifteen to twenty minutes of sun exposure with as much of your skin exposed as possible can generate up to 20,000 IU!

Also, sunlight provides a higher-quality form of vitamin D than you can get from a supplement. When the sunlight hits your skin, cholesterol in your skin becomes oxidized with sulfur, acting as an antioxidant that helps reduce the chance of sunburn. But it also synthesizes vitamin D3 sulfate, which, unlike the vitamin D3 found in supplements, is water soluble. This means it can travel freely in the blood without being packaged into an LDL particle. This is important because it builds a stronger immune system as the sulfates keep your protein matrix healthy and help guard them against microbes. The result is more benefit for protecting against a variety of problems, including inflammation and cancer. Oral vitamin D is less bioavailable and has reduced benefits compared to the natural vitamin D3 sulfate that your body creates from the sun.

So get outside and get some sun exposure each day, and then find some shade or take cover under an umbrella instead of applying sunscreen.

EAT THE RIGHT FOODS

Eating the right foods—and, more importantly, the right amounts of fat, protein, and carbohydrate—can be the biggest factor in reversing the health problems we see all too often today. Food is the substrate that nourishes and rebuilds all the cells in our bodies. Giving your body the right foods is critical to building strong, healthy cells.

A huge component of properly fueling your body is reducing your carbohydrate intake, which helps lower insulin and enables your body to utilize more stored fat. You also must get the right amount of protein each day to ensure that your body can build and repair cells.

We discuss the proper foods to eat on a well-formulated ketogenic diet in much more detail in Chapter 4. For now, just remember that when you give your body the right kinds of fuel, it will reward you with health and longevity.

chapter 3

How Our Bodies Work

The human body is an incredibly complex system, with hundreds of inputs, outputs, and feedback loops that coordinate to sustain life. There are lots of signaling mechanisms (hormones, neurotransmitters, and cytokines) that communicate and control many different processes. Understanding how this system works—and ultimately how it fails—is an important part of understanding why the ketogenic lifestyle can be so important for health and longevity.

The following figure is a complete diagram of the body's metabolic pathways.

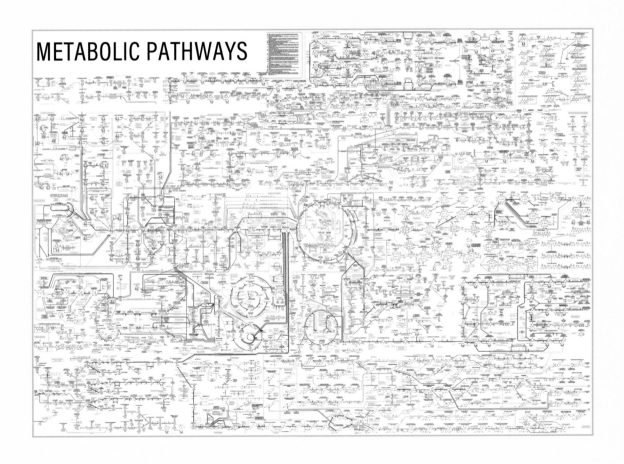

METABOLIC PATHWAYS

Source: biochemical-pathways.com

Many signals, feedback loops, enzymatic processes, and other processes work together to keep you alive. When we look at maps like the one shown in the figure, we are amazed that all these pieces can work together seamlessly—that is, they work seamlessly when we give our bodies the proper inputs. To give you an idea of how complex these metabolic pathways are, the next figure shows lipid (fatty acid) metabolism.

FATTY ACID METABOLISM

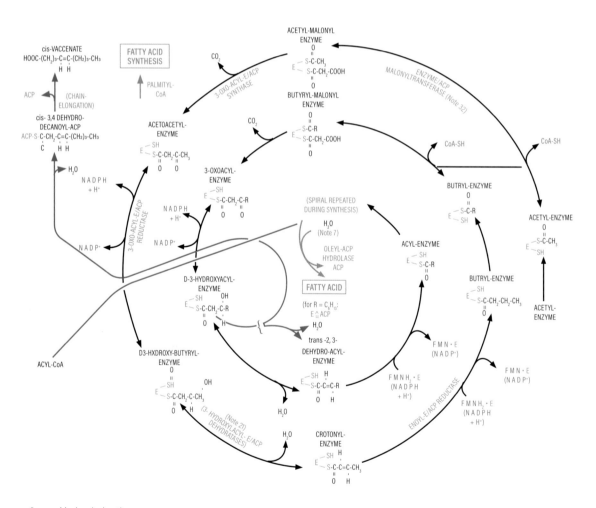

Source: biochemical-pathways.com

Our bodies are very efficient engines. Our bodies are like cars with huge gas tanks. During lean times, when food is scarce, we use stored fuel from our fat storage. Fuel is stored in our fat cells to supply the engine between fill-ups. As with a gasoline engine, you don't want to supply your engine with too much fuel, or you will damage the engine. Our fuel lines (blood vessels) are tightly regulated so that there is never an excess of fuel in the line.

However, unlike cars, our bodies can run on several different fuel sources or substrates that are capable of making adenosine triphosphate (ATP, or cellular energy). These fuel sources are alcohol, ketones (beta-hydroxybutyrate), protein, glucose (sugar), carbohydrates (sugar), and non-esterified fatty acids (NEFA, which are also called free fatty acids—FFA—or just fats).

In this chapter, we look at how metabolism works and how each fuel source is used and prioritized.

METABOLIC FUELS

This section describes the fuels on which our bodies can run. Each burns in different ways and has different effects on the body. Let's take a look at each of these fuels and break down their metabolic pathways.

ALCOHOL

Although alcohol is a source of fuel, your body has no way to store it, so alcohol must be completely burned off before your body can start using other fuels. We will discuss this in more detail later in this chapter in the section titled "Oxidative Priority."

KETONES

Ketones are produced by the liver and are made from free fatty acids. Like alcohol, the body has no storage capability for ketones. Ketones must either be used or excreted (through the urine as acetoacetate or through the breath as acetone). Ketones take oxidative priority as a fuel source over carbohydrates, which means that they are burned when ketones are high and before glucose is used as a fuel.[1] (We discuss exogenous ketones and MCT oils in Chapter 7.) Having both high ketones and high glucose can be a fuel storage nightmare that leads to weight gain.

ALCOHOLISM & A1C LEVELS

Alcoholics actually have very low A1c levels, in the fours. (Read more about A1c levels in Chapter 2.) These low levels don't mean people with alcoholism are healthy—far from it. But it shows how aggressively alcohol demands immediate use because there is no way to store it. When an alcoholic has constantly raised blood alcohol levels, the body aggressively drives down glucose and fat in the blood to keep the fuel supply in the bloodstream in check, which means all this glucose or fat goes right into storage (as glycogen or stored body fat).

There are three types of ketone bodies:

- **Beta-hydroxybutyrate (BHB):** BHB is the main ketone body used for fuel in our cells.

- **Acetoacetate:** BHB and acetoacetate live in a reversible equilibrium and can transform back and forth as needed. Excess or unused acetoacetate can be excreted through the urine.

- **Acetone:** Acetoacetate can also be turned into acetone. But once it is, it cannot be turned back into acetoacetate. Acetone is mostly a waste product of ketone production that is excreted through the breath.

GLUCOSE

Glucose is one of the two primary fuel sources for the body. (FFA is the other.) Your body can store about 1,200 to 2,000 calories of glucose (as glycogen) in your muscles and liver.

Glucose is the fuel source that most of us grew up using. A high-carbohydrate diet (the typical American diet) requires you to eat every couple of hours and ensures that you remain in sugar-burning mode most of the time. However, glucose is intended to be a short-term fuel for which the body has just a small storage tank. Glucose from your diet (carbohydrates) enters your bloodstream first. From there, three things can happen:

- It can be used as fuel for your brain, muscles, and other cells.

- It can be put into storage as glycogen in muscle or the liver.

- It can be turned into triglyceride and stored as fat.

Glucose can go into use (as fuel for the brain, muscles, and so on), but very little is needed at any given moment, especially if you're sitting on the couch after a meal. After all, a normal blood sugar level for an adult is just 4 grams (1 teaspoon) of glucose in your entire volume of blood! The average American today eats more than 300 grams of carbohydrates a day, which equals about 75 teaspoons![2] Worse still, the dietary guidelines of the American Diabetes Association (ADA) say that a diabetic should get 250 to 325 grams of carbohydrates a day![3] Putting 300 grams of carbohydrates into someone who is already insulin resistant and has trouble using carbohydrates when the blood wants only 4 grams at any given time is just crazy.

BURNING GLUCOSE VERSUS BURNING FAT

Think again about the size of the body's fuel tank. You need about 2,000 calories to run 20 miles. Glucose-burners "hit a wall" at about the 18- to 20-mile mark of a marathon because their bodies have been depleted of stored glycogen; the tank is empty. Until you're keto-adapted, you can't quickly switch from burning glucose to burning fat, so your body forces you to stop because it is running out of fuel.

Most of this excess glucose goes into storage in your muscle, liver, or fat cells. But your body has the ability to store glucose as glycogen for only about 1,400 to 2,000 calories, depending on how much muscle mass you have. This is equal to about 350 to 500 grams of glycogen, which is enough for ninety to 120 minutes of exercise. Unless you just finished running a marathon, you won't have anywhere near that much glycogen storage available. When your glycogen storage is full, the extra glucose is turned into triglycerides (through glycolysis and fatty acid synthesis), and triglycerides are stored in adipose tissue (body fat).

FREE FATTY ACIDS

Non-esterified fatty acids (NEFA) or free fatty acids (FFA)—also known as body fat—are the body's biggest source of fuel. The storage capacity is theoretically unlimited. Even very lean athletes have 20,000 or more calories stored in their fat cells. Obese people can have hundreds of thousands of calories stored.

The body stores fat as triglycerides in your fat cells. A triglyceride molecule is made up of three FFA molecules linked together by one glycerol molecule. This process of using FFA for fuel is shown in the FFA metabolism figure earlier in this chapter (see page 50). The large spiral loop in the figure depicts fat flux, which moves fat in and out of storage in fat cells. We discuss fat flux in more detail later in this chapter, beginning on page 61.

PROTEIN

Protein is primarily a body-repair substrate; it is broken into amino acids that are used to build and repair lean mass (muscles, organs, and bones). Protein can also be used as a fuel in very limited quantities. Converting protein to be used for fueling cells is a very energy-intensive process, and the body really only does it as a last resort when you're not consuming other, more efficient fuels (such as glucose and fat). There is also a limited storage capacity for protein—the body can store only about 360 to 480 calories' worth.[4]

THERMIC EFFECT OF FOOD

The thermic effect of food (TEF) is another thing to consider when evaluating different fuel sources. The thermic effect of food refers to how much energy your body needs to use to digest and deal with different macronutrients. Each macro has a different TEF:

- Protein is a whopping 25 percent.
- Alcohol is about 15 percent.
- Carbohydrate is about 8 percent.
- Fat and ketones are only about 3 percent.

This means that for every 100 calories of fat you eat, you end up with a net of 97 calories because of the energy needed to digest it. For every 100 calories of protein you eat, you end up with a net of just 75 calories because using protein (protein synthesis) is an energy-intensive process. It takes a lot of energy for the body to break down protein into amino acids to be used by the body.

THERMIC EFFECT OF FOOD (TEF)

ENERGY SOURCE	TEF	CALORIES CONSUMED	RESULTING CALORIES
Alcohol	15%	100	85
Ketones	3%	100	97
Protein	25%	100	75
Carbohydrates	8%	100	92
Fat	3%	100	97

When you're trying to lose weight, net calorie count is important because certain macronutrients are more beneficial for weight loss because of the energy needed to utilize and digest them. Higher TEF raises your BMR (basal metabolic rate, or the calories you burn throughout the day).

As an example, if you drink a 400-calorie bulletproof coffee (coffee with added butter, MCT oil, and cream), you end up with 388 effective calories in your body. If you eat a 400-calorie steak, you end up with only 300 calories.

OXIDATIVE PRIORITY

Let's discuss how each of the fuel types is used and the order in which they are used. These are both important aspects of our metabolism that lead to the reasons metabolism fails when we don't feed the body properly.

As we've mentioned, our bodies have five different fuel sources: alcohol, ketones, protein, carbohydrates (glucose), and fat. In a normal state (without calories coming into the diet) your body tightly controls the fuel in the blood supply (ketones, glucose, and FFA). During a state of rest, glucose is normally kept at about 80 mg/dl (about 4 grams of glucose in your entire blood volume). Ketones (if you're keto-adapted) can vary. If you have been keto-adapted for several months, your ketones typically will be in the 0.3 to 1.0 mmol/L range. The longer you are keto-adapted the more efficient your body gets at utilizing ketones so fewer are left in the blood. A keto-adapted person can have anywhere from about 0.3 to 5.0 mmol/L in blood ketones. FFA also varies. If you are keto-adapted and at rest, your FFA should be about 1 gram (or 9 calories) or so in blood volume, which is not that much fuel at any given moment. At rest, the total of all the fuels equals maybe 30 calories of energy in your entire blood volume.

When we eat, our bodies have an established process for dealing with each type of fuel. The food you eat gets processed in the GI tract and is sent into the bloodstream. When you eat a 500-calorie meal, there is a lot of fuel going into the bloodstream compared to the 30 calories or so you might normally have circulating in the blood. Your body needs to deal with this fuel so that you don't have an oversupply of fuel in the bloodstream.

To process the fuel, your body first shuts off lipolysis (the process of adding FFA to the blood) so your blood isn't overloaded with fuel. In other words, when you eat, your body stops adding fuel to your blood from storage. Then your body uses oxidative priority to return your blood's fuel levels to normal by processing the fuel in order of priority; it starts with the highest priority fuel: alcohol. Once that fuel is processed, your body processes the second highest priority fuel and continues to move down the line of priority until all fuels are processed. The figure shows this oxidative priority for your body's fuel sources.[5]

OXIDATIVE PRIORITY

Meal Input	Alcohol	Exogenous Ketones	Protein	Carbohydrate	Fat
Oxidative Priority	1	2	3	4	5
Storage System	–	–	Limited [plasma AA]/tissue	Blood [glucose], glycogen	Adipose (fat)
Storage Capacity	Zero	Zero	360–480 calories	1,200–2,000 calories	Unlimited
Postprandial [Blood]					
DIT [Thermogensis] (4–6 hours after meal)	15%		25%	8%	3%

Oxidative priority takes the following order:

- **Alcohol:** Alcohol not only has the number-one position in priority—meaning it must be dealt with before any other fuel gets attention—but it also has no storage capacity. This lack of storage capacity makes alcohol a toxic fuel source. The body must burn it all off—or remove it from the blood—before moving on to deal with other fuels. This is one reason alcohol can lead to weight gain. While your body deals with alcohol, the other fuels from your food are stored, which can lead to massive weight gain.

- **Ketones:** If ketones are elevated by exogenous ketones or MCT oil, your body also needs to deal with that fuel before it can get back to burning fat from your fat stores. Remember, the ultimate goal for fat loss is to use the fat from your fat stores for fuel. Each time you eat, your body stops using fat stores for fuel until all the fuel from the meal is used or stored. Then the body can go back to using the fuel stores (fat) for fuel.

- **Protein:** Protein is the body's building blocks for making and repairing lean body mass, such as when you break down muscle during a workout or when your body is repairing or replacing damaged body tissue and bone. If you take in very large amounts of protein—something that is hard to do—your body must burn excess protein that's not needed for repairing and building. Your body has little or no storage for protein. But the body would rather burn FFA or glucose. Glucose takes only two ATP (units of energy) to be broken down into fuel for the cells. Turning protein into glucose (through a process called gluconeogenesis) takes six ATP and then another two ATP to turn this into cellular energy. This is very inefficient.

- **Carbohydrate:** Carbohydrate is one of the body's two preferred fuel sources (the other is fat). If you don't drink, don't take exogenous ketones, and keep your protein moderate, your body is ready to burn glucose. Almost every cell in the body can burn glucose or fat. However, the body also likes to keep blood glucose in a tight window—70 to 120 mg/dl, which is about 1 teaspoon of glucose (4 grams of carbs) in your entire blood volume. If you are eating a large Salted Caramel Truffle Blizzard that contains 188 grams of carbohydrates, you are getting 47 teaspoons of glucose in your blood when the body only wants 1 teaspoon. Your body has only about 1,200 to at most 2,000 calories of storage space for glucose (300 to 500 grams). And that much space is available only if you have just run a marathon and completely depleted your glycogen stores. Your body will need a long time to store and use that glucose, so every bit of fat that was also in that frosty treat (some might have 67 grams) will get stored in your fat cells. (We talk more about this later.) The main idea here is that you want to keep the carbohydrates as low as you can so your body can get to burning fat for fuel.

- **Fat:** The last fuel on the oxidative priority is fat. Oxidative priority makes the concepts of a well-formulated ketogenic lifestyle obvious. Don't drink any alcohol; don't take any exogenous ketones; eat moderate amounts of protein (just enough to satisfy your body's lean mass needs); and limit carbohydrates as much as you can. Then eat just enough fat to keep your hormones happy. This clears the oxidative priority and allows the body to burn fat and utilize stored fat for fuel. Here's why fat is the body's preferred fuel source:

- **Fat is dense.** Fat contains about 9 calories per gram versus 4 calories per gram in protein and carbs.
- **Our bodies have a nearly unlimited capacity for storing fat.** Even very lean athletes with 12 percent body fat can have 20,000 calories stored in their fat cells, which is more than ten times what is available in glucose (glycogen). Someone carrying 100 pounds of body fat has more than 408,000 calories stored. This is how our ancestors survived long cold winters and lean months when hunting and gathering food was difficult. They filled up their fat stores in summer and used that stored fat in the winter.

LIPOLYSIS

Our adipose tissue (stored body fat) has many fat molecules (triglycerides) in each cell or adipocyte. Think of a fat cell as a storage compartment with a bunch of triglyceride molecules stuffed into it. Each triglyceride is a molecule made of three FFA molecules and one glycerol molecule (95 percent fat and 5 percent glucose).

The process of lipolysis is when the triglyceride molecule has the glycerol cleaved (separated) from the three FFA molecules; the triglyceride molecule is then sent into the bloodstream. Interestingly, this glycerol is what helps us attain a ketogenic state. Three glycerol molecules make one glucose molecule. As your body burns fat, it also creates glucose that can fuel parts of the brain and other body parts that cannot run on FFA. This is actually a large source of the gluconeogenesis that occurs when you are keto-adapted.

The FFA molecules are fuel and can be directly burned by muscle and other tissues. When you are keto-adapted and following a well-formulated ketogenic diet, you are burning lots of FFAs from the food you eat and from your fat stores (which means fat loss). For fat loss, you want to burn as much as possible from your fat stores.

A 1928 study titled "Studies on the Metabolism of Eskimos" demonstrates the extent to which the body is able to make glucose from body fat (glycerol). In this study, Peter Heinbecker tested an Eskimo woman who was breastfeeding a baby.[6] When she was tested, she had eaten nothing for three and a half days. She was excreting both glucose and galactose in her breast milk, but her glycogen stores were used up after three and a half days of fasting. So where was the sugar coming from? Her fat stores. She had an RQ (respiratory quotient) of 0.45! An RQ of 0.8 is a mixed diet of fat, protein, and carbs. An RQ of 1.0 is a diet composed mainly of carbs. An RQ of 0.7 is a diet composed mainly of fat. This mother was so deeply burning fat and generating glycerol that she was able to meet not only her own body's demand for glucose, but also the extra demand needed to produce breast milk.

In fact, when you are keto-adapted, your muscles become more insulin resistant (called physiological insulin resistance)—and this is not a bad thing. Your muscles prefer to burn FFA for fuel. Lower insulin levels allow lipolysis to occur, making more FFA available to be used as fuel. Muscles burn FFA while rejecting glucose. Because your muscles reject glucose (when you are keto-adapted) that glucose is used by the brain and other body parts that can't use FFA as fuel. This process explains why some people who are just starting to get keto-adapted can see higher fasting glucose levels. The muscles aren't using glucose as their main fuel source anymore, which leaves more glucose in the bloodstream. After a few weeks, the blood glucose levels out as the body becomes more keto-adapted.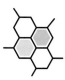

Lipolysis isn't just about weight loss; it's also about healing. As discussed in Chapter 2, inflamed and overstuffed fat cells are what start the cycle toward insulin resistance and disrupted hormone signaling. The most important thing you can do to start the healing process (and reverse insulin resistance) is to get lipolysis going to shrink the fat cells enough to restore normal insulin response and signaling. Lipolysis is necessary for weight loss and to enable healing from metabolic issues.

What stops lipolysis? Insulin. Even a tiny rise in insulin (even from eating fat) will stop lipolysis because your body allows only so much fuel to be in your bloodstream at any moment. When you eat—and thus fuel enters the bloodstream—your body immediately stops adding fuel to your blood from your fat stores; in other words,

HOMEOSTATIC MODEL ASSESSMENT OF INSULIN RESISTANCE (HOMA-IR)

If your fasting glucose has increased due to physiological insulin resistance, how do you determine whether it is an issue? You need to look at glucose and insulin together. The HOMA-IR model (Homeostatic Model Assessment of Insulin Resistance) can give you the answer. HOMA-IR = (glucose x insulin) / 405 (in mg/dL) or HOMA-IR = (glucose x insulin) / 22.5) (in mmol/L). This tells you if you have higher glucose but much lower insulin, which results in a lower number—the lower the number, the better. When you are a sugar-burner and both glucose and insulin are high, you have a problem. A HOMA-IR of 1.0 or less means you are insulin sensitive; 1.9 or above is early insulin resistance; and 2.9 or higher is significant insulin resistance.

GLUCOSE, INSULIN, TRIGLYCERIDE, AND LEPTIN RESPONSE TO INGESTED CARBOHYDRATE, PROTEIN, AND FAT[7]

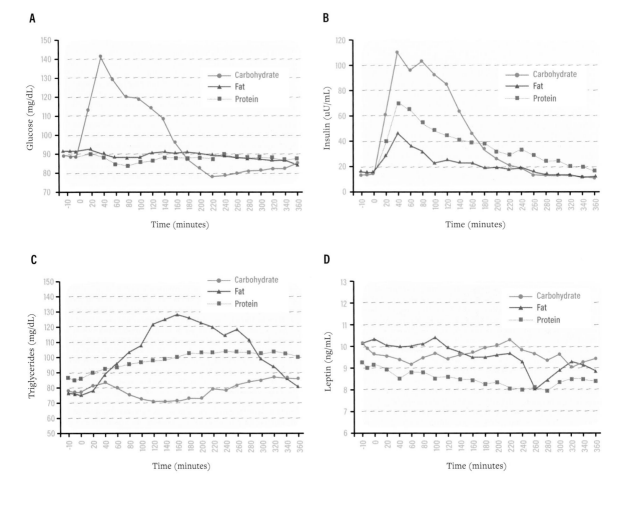

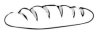

Carbs Raise Insulin Levels

All fuels increase insulin, though some fuels—carbohydrates—raise insulin more than others. However, even fat increases insulin a small amount—enough to shut off lipolysis. Insulin is boosted by increased carb intake because your body tries to prevent an oversupply of fuel in your blood. If your body is sending fat from the fat stores into the blood while fat is coming in through the digestive tract, your body stops burning fat from your fat stores, which means lipolysis stops.

lipolysis stops. Once lipolysis stops, your body starts using and/or storing the fuel coming in instead of using the fuel stored in your fat cells. As you can see in the figure opposite, every fuel that comes into the bloodstream from the diet affects insulin.

As you can see in the top-right chart of the figure, insulin is raised when any macronutrient is ingested. Carbohydrates have the largest insulin response, followed by protein and then fat. Exogenous ketones are not shown but would likely have an effect on insulin that is similar to fat. However, there is still enough of a rise in insulin from ingesting fat to stop lipolysis and cause your body to turn to storing fat instead of using your fat stores.

Fat storage or fat used from fat cells is highly dependent on insulin. Let's look closer at how fat flux works.

FAT FLUX

The FFA metabolism figure on page 50 shows the section of our metabolic pathways that represents lipolysis, which looks like a large spiral; this spiral represents fat flux.

There are two inputs into a fat cell:

- The first input comes from the dietary carbohydrates that are stored in the fat cells when excess carbohydrates are converted into fat and stored; this process is called *de novo lipogenesis*. Many people think this is where most of their stored fat comes from. However, only about 5 percent of the stored fat comes from carbohydrates.[8] When your carb intake is high, oxidative priority forces your body to store all the fat coming in with the carbs while your body is busy storing and burning those excess carbs.

- The second input is from unused fats (triglycerides) that are being put back into storage.

The one way fat leaves a fat cell is by lipolysis. Lipolysis allows fatty acids to enter the bloodstream and is the output of fat flux. Think of fat flux like a bucket with a tap and valve on the bottom. The two inputs (de novo lipogenesis and triglycerides) are like pouring water into the bucket, which causes the amount of water in the bucket to increase. If the valve at the bottom of the bucket is open—lipolysis in this example—some of that water exits, which reduces the total amount of water in the bucket. The inputs create fat gain, and the output (lipolysis) creates fat loss. To lose fat, your body needs to create a net outward flux, meaning your body needs to send more fat out than is going back into the fat cells.

During lipolysis, you have more fat from your fat stores in your bloodstream than your cells need at any given moment. This process is believed to be in preparation for a sudden burst of activity—say, running from a hungry lion. This additional fuel is available in case there is a sudden need for extra fuel.

However, once this fuel (FFA) enters the bloodstream, there are two paths it can take:

- **Used for fuel:** It can be used for fuel in the muscles and other tissues.
- **Sent back into storage:** If it doesn't get used for fuel, it gets sent to the liver to be packaged back up into a triglyceride molecule (called esterification). This triglyceride is then packaged into a VLDL particle and sent back into fat storage. The following figure shows this process.[9]

FAT FLUX

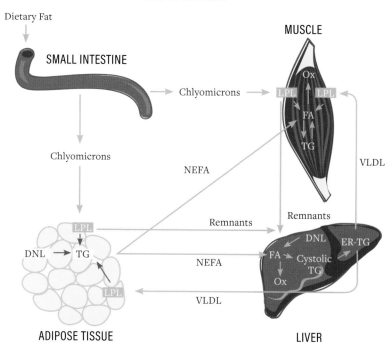

LIVER

CO$_2$
(muscle)

ADIPOSE TISSUE

The figure above doesn't show dietary fat, but the following figure shows the dietary fat part of the cycle.[10]

LIPID EXCHANGE

The process looks like this:

1. Dietary fat is transported from your small intestine in chylomicrons (carriers that take dietary fats from the intestines to other body parts) to be used as fuel in tissue, but its primary destination is storage in your fat cells (adipose tissue).

2. When insulin is low and your body needs fuel, the fat cell cleaves or strips the glycerol from the triglyceride, leaving three FFA molecules and one glycerol molecule.

3. FFA leaving your fat cells stays as FFA and is bound to albumin to be transported in your blood to your muscles and other tissues as available fuel. This is one of the primary fuel sources for your body when energy isn't coming in through your diet.

4. Whatever FFA isn't used as fuel makes its way to the liver where it is packaged (esterified) into a triglyceride molecule.

5. From there, it is packaged into VLDL particles and sent back into circulation to be used as fuel in tissues or, more commonly, redeposited into fat cells.

There is a constant flux of fat in and out of the fat cells. Also, as described in Chapter 2, if the fat cells get overstuffed and inflamed, this fat flux breaks down because the overstuffed fat cells are resisting insulin. As more fat comes in through your diet or in VLDL particles from your liver, it can't be stored. Also, fat accumulates in the blood, liver, and pancreas, causing a metabolic breakdown. To lose fat and reverse metabolic damage, you need more fat to come out of the fat cells than is going in.

DO CALORIES MATTER?

At this point, you might be wondering if this is just the old calories in, calories out advice. We are definitely not saying a calorie is a calorie. The different foods and macronutrients we eat have vastly different effects on our hormones and metabolisms. (We discuss hormones in detail in Chapter 5.)

The keto diet doesn't rely solely on the calories in, calories out model because the makeup of those calories matters due to the hormonal response to different macronutrients in the body. Unfortunately, there are two schools of thought in the keto community—one that says calories and fat intake don't matter, and the other that says calories and fat do matter. We are in the second camp, and we believe calories definitely do matter. If you eat 5,000 calories a day of any food (even just fat) you will not lose weight. But hormones matter, too. They both matter.

When eating keto, you are trying to find an in-between point. Calories matter, but the makeup of those calories also matters. The most important factor of the makeup of those calories is the balance of fat, protein, and carbs and how each affects insulin levels. As we discussed earlier in this chapter, any rise in insulin stops lipolysis, so you want to eat foods that create the smallest rise in insulin so that you burn in-body fat for fuel (lipolysis). There is also the concept of limiting the fuels in the oxidative priority to more quickly get back to fat burning. That means consuming no alcohol, no exogenous ketones, and little to no carbohydrate so that your body goes about synthesizing protein, fat-burning, and fat-storing. Being keto-adapted helps keep fat flux going and keeps you burning fat for fuel.

There's also the impact on other hormones, such as ghrelin and leptin, that send an "I'm full" signal to your brain. Empty carbs like refined sugar don't send that signal, so we can eat them in large volumes and still never feel full. Protein, and to some extent fat, causes your body to send a full signal much sooner. It is very hard to overeat when eating protein. For most people, a 16-ounce steak would be difficult to finish. That 16-ounce steak represents about 900 calories (even less when you consider the thermic effect of food), and yet most people would feel full all day on that much protein. However, if you eat a 1,000-calorie milkshake containing more than 100 grams of sugar, you will likely be hungry again in two to three hours when insulin overcorrects and your blood sugar drops too low.

Calories and hormones matter; a ketogenic diet is so powerful because it can be used to address both. A ketogenic diet keeps our hormones in balance, which helps us to feel full longer and eliminates cravings—and we can do these things while eating fewer calories.

MORE ABOUT ALCOHOL

We once had a client who told us he had to have a few glasses of wine in the evening so that ketones would be present when he tested his levels in the morning. He said if he didn't drink alcohol, ketones were not present. Our first thought was, "Um, what?" But it turns out, he was right.

The truth is that alcohol doesn't help you get into ketosis; if anything, alcohol will hold you back from your goals. As you might remember from our discussion of oxidative priority, alcohol cannot be stored, and it is first in line to be processed, ahead of protein, carbs, fat, and so on. Your body must burn off alcohol before it can deal with any other fuel or get back to lipolysis.

ALCOHOL FACTS

When people go on a diet, they often choose the "light" versions of their favorite alcoholic beverages in order to save a few calories. However, calories are only one small piece of the puzzle. After only two alcoholic beverages, fat metabolism is reduced by as much as 73 percent. This scary fact shows that the primary effect of alcohol on the body is to stop the body from using fat stores for energy.

Alcohol is converted in the body to a substance called *acetate*. Unlike a car that uses only one supply of fuel, the body can draw from carbohydrates, fats, ketones, and proteins for energy. When your blood acetate levels rise, your body uses acetate instead of fat. To make matters worse, the more alcohol you drink, the more you tend to eat, and unfortunately, drinking makes your liver work to convert the alcohol to acetate, which means that the foods you consume at the same time will be converted to extra fat on your body. If that isn't bad enough, alcohol also stimulates appetite and decreases testosterone levels for up to twenty-four hours, and it increases estrogen by 300 percent. The infamous "beer belly" is really just an "estrogen belly." Biochemically, the higher your estrogen level, the more readily you absorb alcohol and the more slowly you break it down.

Alcohol affects every organ of the body, with the most dramatic effect being upon the liver. The liver cells normally prefer fatty acids as fuel; the liver packages excess fatty acids as triglycerides to be stored back in fat cells (fat flux). However, when alcohol is present, the liver cells are forced to metabolize the alcohol first, while allowing large amounts of fatty acids to accumulate. Alcohol metabolism permanently changes liver cell structure, which impairs the liver's ability to metabolize fats and can lead to fatty liver disease.

Alcohol and sugar addiction go hand in hand. We have heavy hearts for people who have food addictions because, unlike alcohol, food is unavoidable; we need it for survival. Many people claim that it is impossible to be addicted to sugar, but research has proven that when people binge on carbs (which are sugar molecules hooked together in long chains) and then restrict those carbs, the body creates an endogenous (internal) opioid. This endogenous opioid is similar to the chemicals released when people legally or illegally use opioid drugs. PET and CT scans of food addicts show that food lights up the same areas of the brain that are lighted in people who are drug addicts. What we find really interesting is that "carb addicts" carry the same D2 dopamine receptor (a gene that identifies addiction); this fact suggests that, biochemically, food addictions are very similar to addictions to narcotics. A lot of our clients who are members of Overeaters Anonymous tell us that they started consuming carbs and sugar just as if they were alcohol.

American society views alcoholism as a problem but views carb and sugar consumption as "normal"—as a part of the typical American diet. This isn't the case everwhere in the world, though. We had one client who lived and worked in England for ten years. While she was there, her company paid for her to seek treatment for her sugar addiction. British physicians recognized her problem and how it was affecting her work. However, now that she has returned to the U.S., she is seen as normal.

We want you to know that there are ways to help your brain chemistry. You do not have to suffer from a food or alcohol addiction. Sugar (and alcohol) blocks serotonin receptors, which leads to more cravings for carbs and alcohol. Serotonin comes from the intestinal tract, not the brain. To correct this problem, we recommend *Bifidobacteria*, a probiotic found in food sources such as naturally fermented vegetables and organ meats. However, because people tend not to eat enough of these foods, we also suggest a supplement to increase serotonin. Seventy percent of your immune system starts in your gut. We believe that *Bifidobacteria* is one of the best things to take if you are depressed or dealing with cravings.

HOW TO GET INTO A NEGATIVE FAT FLUX (LOSE FAT)

You lose weight and heal from metabolic issues by achieving a negative fat flux. To do so, you need to start shrinking your fat cells, which allows you to lose fat and restore insulin signaling.

The best way to get into a negative fat flux is to clear out your body's oxidative priority as much as you can. This means

- Eliminating alcohol
- Staying away from exogenous ketones
- Eating enough protein to meet your lean mass needs
- Eating very few carbs
- Eating only enough fat to keep cravings down and keep making healthy hormones

Altering your diet in this way keeps insulin to a minimum and helps your body get back to burning body fat for fuel more quickly. You use dietary fat as a control switch for lipolysis. The more dietary fat you eat, the less body fat you use for fuel and the more lipolysis is shut off. Less dietary fat means that lipolysis is running more and you are using more body fat for fuel (which leads to fat loss).

A low-carb, moderate-protein, and moderate-fat diet—in other words, a well-formulated ketogenic diet—allows your body to continue making healthy hormones and absorbing fat-soluble vitamins while remaining in fat-burning mode. This diet creates a negative fat flux, helps you lose fat, and keeps your hormones in check so you don't experience spikes and crashes in insulin and hunger. The keto diet allows you to take in fewer calories while forcing your body to use more body fat for fuel. It also keeps your body in fat-burning mode so that it can easily switch from burning dietary fat to burning body fat for fuel.

In Chapter 4, we discuss what a well-formulated ketogenic diet is and how you can use it to get into a negative fat flux.

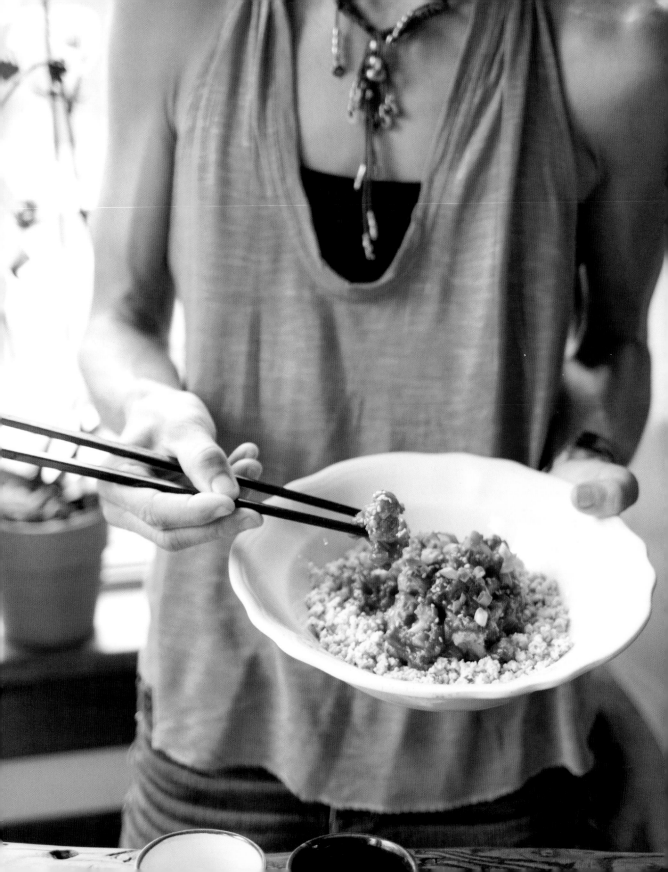

chapter 4

What Is a Well-Formulated Ketogenic Diet?

The human body is an amazing machine. It is complex to a degree that we are only beginning to understand. You are filled with systems and feedback loops that control your body's functions and reactions to external signals (food, light, nutrients, and so on). In this chapter, we discuss how to design the inputs so that you lose weight and heal.

In Chapter 3, we explain that whether you lose weight and heal depends largely on getting your body into a negative fat flux, which means burning more body fat than you store. There are a few ways in which a well-formulated ketogenic diet helps you get into a negative fat flux.

MACRONUTRIENT TARGETS

Getting your macronutrients, or "macros," right is a big component of a well-formulated ketogenic diet. Also, eating organic, whole foods is helpful for reducing the load on your liver and for detoxing. This is why we advocate a whole-foods approach to a ketogenic diet. Let's go through the basic components of a well-formulated ketogenic diet.

CARBOHYDRATES

The most important thing for getting into ketosis is getting your macros right, and the most important one to get right is carbohydrates. Getting your carbs to fewer than 30 grams a day (20 grams for those with metabolic issues) will ensure that you are in ketosis.

Your carbohydrate tolerance depends on a lot of factors. Some athletes can eat up to 50 grams of carbs a day and stay in ketosis because they are very active. Other people who have metabolic damage need to stay at fewer than 20 grams a day.

We use total carbs to make things easier and because some fiber carbs (such as inulin) can affect blood sugar and hold you back. Counting total carbs eliminates this problem and ensures that you are in ketosis.

PROTEIN

The second most important component of a well-formulated ketogenic diet is to hit your protein target. You want to get to your protein goal every day; if you can't hit it each day, you want to at least average out to your goal over the course of a week. That means you might eat more protein one day and less the next; the goal is to have enough protein over the course of the week so that your average equals your goal target.

Protein builds and repairs your lean mass (muscles, soft tissues, and many other critical body parts). We know that probably the most important thing for vitality and longevity is not to lose lean mass as we age. Getting adequate protein helps ensure that your lean mass doesn't decrease too much. Low-protein approaches are damaging over time because you slowly lose lean mass, which is not what you want to have happen as you age.

To find your protein goal, multiply your lean body mass (your total weight minus your body fat) by 0.8. For example, if you weigh 180 pounds and have 40 percent body fat, you have 108 pounds of lean mass (180 x 0.6). So your protein goal would be 86 grams a day (0.8 x 108).

FAT

If you get your carbs and protein right, then, as Luis Villasenor of KetoGains.com likes to say, "Fat is a lever." This means that you can think of fat as a lever that regulates fat flux. When you raise

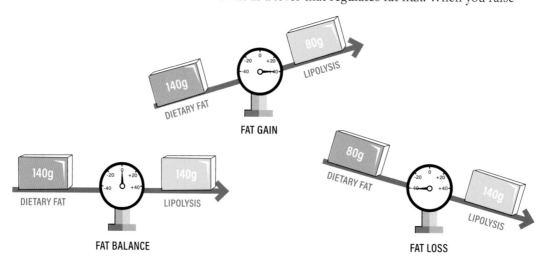

dietary fat (move the lever higher), less body fat is used for fuel. When you lower the lever (reduce dietary fat), more body fat is used for fuel (more negative fat flux). Fat is our best source of energy, and when you are keto-adapted, your body can use body fat and dietary fat equally well. If weight loss and healing are your goals, you need to use more body fat for fuel!

FORMULATING A KETOGENIC DIET FOR WEIGHT LOSS AND HEALING

On a well-formulated ketogenic diet, you are primarily burning fat for fuel. However, to lose fat and reverse metabolic damage, your body needs to use more body fat than dietary fat. This doesn't mean you get zero dietary fat. You can try adding some protein-sparing modified fasting (PSMF) to break a stall or increase fat loss, but even then you are getting enough fat (40 to 50 grams) to fuel proper hormone development and nutrient absorption (fat-soluble vitamins like A, D, E, and K). We cover PSMF later in this chapter.

However, in the first couple of weeks after switching to a keto lifestyle, you might need to add more fat because your body isn't efficient at burning fat (and ketones) yet. Adding more fat to your diet can help with energy, focus, moods, and the like.

There are three stages or phases of a well-formulated ketogenic lifestyle. Let's look at these phases and what you can expect with each one.

PHASE 1: GENERATING ELEVATED BLOOD KETONES

Within the first two to four days of lowering your carb intake to below 20 grams a day, you will start showing elevated blood ketones, which marks the start of your body utilizing nutritional ketosis (and lipolysis) and shifting its primary fuel source to fat. However, you might have issues with energy, moods, headaches, or other common "keto flu" symptoms. To combat the symptoms of keto flu, you first must make sure to keep your water and electrolytes up. When becoming keto-adapted, your kidneys release much of the salt (and associated water) that they hold onto with higher-carb diets. You need to add more water and electrolytes to ensure that you don't get dehydrated. You also might want to reduce your workouts and activity levels during the first couple weeks.

Even though your blood ketones are higher, your body isn't efficient at using them yet. Many people find it helpful to add fat bombs (high-fat, low-carb snacks) in the first couple of weeks. Make a dessert, some deviled eggs, or something similar to have on hand when cravings strike. However, as your hunger declines and your energy increases, eliminate the extra fat to improve your results (burn more body fat for fuel).

The more metabolic damage you have, the longer you will remain in Phase 1. The next phase is where you start seeing your body get better at burning fat as its primary fuel.

 ## PHASE 2: BECOMING KETO-ADAPTED (A TRUE FAT-BURNER)

In this stage, the body and cells get better at utilizing fat as their primary fuel source, which results in fewer cravings, feeling fuller throughout the day, better moods, more restful sleep, and much more energy.

Depending on how metabolically damaged you are, Phase 2 can take anywhere from two to six weeks or more. Most people start feeling the benefits after three to four weeks. When you start feeling results, you should reduce your added snacks and fat bombs to increase the use of body fat for fuel (fat loss).

Becoming keto-adapted takes this long because your body makes a cellular-level change to accommodate burning fat as its primary fuel source. Glucose burns very easily as a fuel; it contains lots of quick energy and needs fewer mitochondria to get all the fuel it needs. Turning free fatty acids (FFA) into fuel takes a bit more effort. When you first make the shift to eating keto, your body's cellular makeup needs to change to accommodate burning large amounts of fat. This process also explains why your energy dips and your workouts suffer in the first couple weeks of going keto.

Your body needs to make more mitochondria to increase its capacity to burn fat for fuel.[1] Mitochondria are the little powerhouses in our cells that turn fuel (FFA, ketones, glucose) into energy (ATP). By increasing the number of mitochondria, your body increases how much fat it can burn at any given time. Studies have shown that athletic performance on a keto diet can equal performance on a high-carbohydrate diet after a two- to four-week adaption period.[2]

During this time, your ketone levels drop because your body is using more FFA directly for fuel instead of turning it into ketones and then using it for fuel. This is an important distinction because the elevated ketone levels in the early stages of keto-adaptation are part of a transitional state in which your body creates more ketones. These additional ketones help fuel your body until it can create more mitochondria so it can burn more FFA directly, which is another reason not to chase ketone levels.

 ## PHASE 3: A DEEPER MITOCHONDRIAL LEVEL OF KETOSIS

In this phase, you start to see even more improvements. We have many clients who start saying things like, "I am just not hungry," and "I can finally keep up with my kids all day!"

After about three or four months of a ketogenic lifestyle, you start to experience how good your body can feel. Those afternoon slumps are gone. Energy is endless. You never have cravings and are almost always satiated. Food becomes an afterthought instead of something you think about all day long.

At this point, your body has increased the number of mitochondria in your cells and is continuing to transform white adipose tissue (WAT or white fat) to brown adipose tissue (BAT or brown fat).[3] BAT is a sort of activated fat—that is, fat cells that contain mitochondria. White fat stores fat; brown fat handles thermoregulation (regulating body temperature). This is an important change that brings many benefits.

This shift to brown fat can reduce your glucose levels. The brown fat starts using glucose to generate heat, which can help keep glucose levels in check and can also lead to you feeling warmer because brown fat generates heat instead of being dormant like white fat. This shift to brown fat also increases your BMR (basal metabolic rate), or the amount of energy your body consumes all day long. Having more brown fat can be a great metabolic advantage.

Also, the longer you are in ketosis, the more cholesterol (substrate) your body has to produce healthy hormones. This additional cholesterol allows your body to shift your hormones to a more natural set point for your body when given enough saturated fat and cholesterol. The balancing of your hormones has many other benefits, including improved fertility, deeper sleep, better moods, and increased mental clarity. Chronic conditions, such as Crohn's disease and irritable bowel syndrome, start to improve because inflammation has decreased. A long-term ketogenic lifestyle has many health benefits, including greater longevity and the reversal of many chronic diseases.

This chart shows why keto is a lifestyle rather than a quick-fix diet. You can't eat keto for a couple of weeks, expect results, and then go back to eating junk. Keto causes a shift in the way your body functions at a cellular level. If you commit to a keto lifestyle, it will continue rewarding you with improvements to your health and how you feel.

PHASE 1

2–3 days

Ketones up 1.0+

Energy ↓

Hunger ↑

Mitochondria same

Fat same

PHASE 2

2–4 weeks or more

Ketones moderate 0.5–2.0

Energy ↑

Hunger ↓

Mitochondria ↑

Fat shifting

PHASE 3

3–4 months or more

Ketones moderate 0.3–1.0

Energy ↑↑

Hunger ↓↓

Mitochondria ↑↑

Fat shifting

Keto Adaptation Phases

1. At the start, ketones rise after two to three days. FFA oxidation increases a little, up to 1.0 or 2.0 mmol. Energy dips, and fasting glucose can float up a bit.

2. After two to four weeks, energy increases and ketones drop to maybe 0.5 to 1.0 mmol. FFA oxidation goes up significantly and fasting glucose levels out.

3. After three to four months, energy continues to rise while ketones drop to maybe 0.3 or 0.5 mmol. FFA oxidation reaches its peak, and fasting glucose lowers (to maybe 85).

A WELL-FORMULATED KETOGENIC DIET

A well-formulated ketogenic diet takes into account all the body's needs:

- It is nutrient-dense.
- It supplies enough protein to preserve lean mass.
- It reduces carbs to ensure that you stay in ketosis.
- It helps you remember that to lose fat, you need to use more stored body fat and less dietary fat (net negative fat flux).

To have a well-formulated ketogenic diet, you need to focus on the things that matter. Eat nutrient-dense animal proteins to get the nutrients you need to hit your protein goals while keeping carbs to a minimum. Then use fat as a lever to increase or reduce fat loss from your fat cells. Keto is pretty easy when you think of it this way! Let's look at an example of a well-formulated keto diet.

Consider a woman who weighs 170 pounds, has 38 percent body fat, and is fairly sedentary. She has about 105 pounds of lean body mass and a basal metabolic rate (BMR, or the number of calories needed to maintain) of about 1,540 calories.

We recommend that this woman consume more fat during her first couple of weeks on a ketogenic diet (especially if she has a lot of metabolic damage) to help with moods, focus, and energy. Her well-formulated macros would be 120 to 130 grams of fat, 84 grams of protein, and 20 grams of carbs for a total of about 1,500 calories. This 1,500-calorie amount is about her BMR level of calories, which will help fuel her body during the first couple weeks; this level of fat also will help fuel her brain while it adapts and gets better at making the fuel on its own. Also, she should make sure to get extra water, sodium, potassium, and magnesium. Good goals are about 4 grams of sodium, 4.5 to 5 grams of potassium, and 400 to 800 milligrams of magnesium. Note that sodium must be added to food and even water if needed. Most people are deficient in magnesium, so adding a supplement is a good idea (400 to 800 milligrams per day). You get a lot of potassium from food (such as red meat), so your need for a supplement depends on how much potassium you get from what you eat and how your body reacts to eating this way. If you start to experience leg cramps, a heart flutter, or other symptoms, you might want to add more electrolytes.

After the woman's cravings subside and her energy increases, she is keto-adapted, and her well-formulated macros would be 90 grams (or less) of fat, 84 grams of protein, and 20 grams of carbs for a total of about 1,200 calories. Now, she is reducing her dietary fat intake to force her body to use more body fat for fuel. If the BMR level dictates that she consume 1,540 calories, the extra fat required is pulled from the fat stores as shown in the chart below (for a day with 90 grams of fat).

Once the woman is keto-adapted, she should start increasing her activity, including incorporating more small movements (taking the stairs, walking to the mailbox, and so on). The longer she has been keto-adapted, she can add strength training, yoga, or other activities. Remember that working out stimulates autophagy (generating new healthy and younger cells) as well as making more mitochondria and lean muscle mass to help you stay strong and have a higher BMR to burn more calories all day long.

When the woman reaches her weight loss and/or healing goals, she increases her fat intake to find her body's maintenance point; her carb and protein intake stay the same. Increasing fat intake while maintaining carb and protein intake can be achieved by adding sauces and dressings to meals or eating snacks or keto treats.

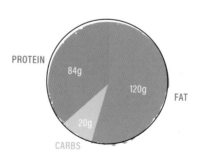

In the first 1 to 4 weeks of going keto

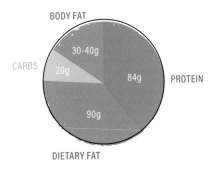

BODY FAT

30-40g

CARBS

20g   84g   PROTEIN

90g

DIETARY FAT

After hunger subsides and
cravings diminish

Breaking down the ketogenic diet into its macronutrient components is easy. Just find your protein goal and hit it each day (or average out to it over the course of a week), keep your carb intake below 20 grams a day, and modulate fat as needed to achieve your particular goals. Keep your water and electrolytes up in the process, and you will do great! Check out Chapter 11 for some super-easy meal plans for a well-formulated ketogenic diet.

FAT IN A KETO DIET

The idea that you need to eat a high-fat diet in order to follow a ketogenic lifestyle is a myth. Adding lots of fat can increase ketone levels, but having high ketone levels isn't the goal. Here are just a few ways to be keto (have elevated ketones):

- Eat 20 grams or less of total carbs.
- Eat nothing (fast) for more than twenty-four hours.
- Eat 20 grams of carbs or less with little to no fat.
- Eat 20 grams of carbs or less with lots of fat.
- Eat only carbs and keep total calorie intake at or below 400 calories a day.
- Eat only protein.
- Eat anything and do insane amounts of exercise (depleting glycogen stores causes ketones to rise).
- Depending on age, don't eat anything for a few hours (see the chart on the next page). Newborns are always in ketosis (when breastfed) and have blood ketones of 0.5 mmol when they're feeding; that rises to 2.0 mmol after only two hours of not eating. A six- to eight-year-old has blood ketones of 0.5 mmol after five to six hours of not eating. Adults see blood ketones of 0.5 after about fourteen hours of not eating.

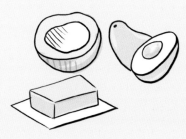

Note that this list doesn't include "fake keto," in which elevated ketones are induced via exogenous ketones or large amounts of MCT oil. You can eat a big bowl of rice covered in MCT oil and show elevated blood ketones, but that meal isn't going to help you reach your weight-loss and health goals.

However, this does demonstrate that eating large amounts of fat is not a requirement for being in ketosis. As described in Chapter 3, you can't eat large amounts of fat if you expect to lose stored fat.

HOURS UNTIL YOU SHOW ELEVATED BLOOD KETONES, BY AGE[4]

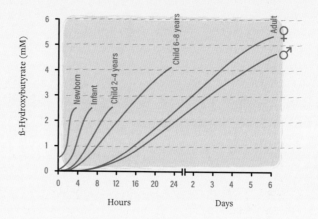

ELECTROLYTES

As we mentioned in our example of a well-formulated ketogenic diet, getting enough electrolytes and water is an important part of becoming keto-adapted, especially in the first few weeks after making the switch to keto. Let's take a deeper look at electrolytes and their benefits.

Sodium

Even if adapting to a keto lifestyle doesn't cause any obvious side effects, you need extra water and sodium. Eliminating packaged foods will likely deplete a lot of the sodium from your diet. The recommended foods for the keto diet don't contain a lot of liquid, so you will want to drink at least half your body weight in ounces of water every day. If you suffer the fierce headaches that some people get when beginning a low-carb diet, add sodium.

Get More Sodium by Drinking Homemade Bone Broth

Our favorite way for clients to get more sodium is to consume homemade bone broth. It is so easy to make—you can even do it in a slow cooker! Bone broth contains sodium as well as a ton of minerals and electrolytes. Commercial broths do not convey these same benefits, as they don't contain all the collagen and minerals found in traditionally prepared bone broth. (However, some companies have started to offer boxed bone broths that have the same healthy benefits as homemade bone broth; Kettle & Fire is one example.) Bone broth takes at least one day to make (and up to three days for ultra-rich broth), but we often make a huge batch in the pot Craig used years ago to make home-brewed beer. (Yes, we have come a long way in our journey!) We freeze the bone broth in small containers, and it keeps for a very long time.

We suggest throwing out your regular table salt and replacing it with a quality mineral-rich sea salt or rock salt. (Celtic sea salt and Himalayan rock salt are good options.) Real salt is essential for electrolyte balance and will give you energy. After a few months of using sea salt or rock salt, you will likely find that table salt has a chemical-like taste.

It's not necessary to use these Celtic or Himalayan salts sparingly, either. These salts are either harvested from ancient sea beds or made by evaporating seawater with a high mineral content. They contain about 70 percent of the sodium in regular salt (which has been refined, bleached, and processed until it is pretty much pure sodium chloride, often with anti-caking agents added). The other 30 percent consists of minerals and micronutrients (including iodine) found in mineral-rich seas. In terms of taste, we greatly prefer these salts to regular salt; they are well worth the extra cost. Do not make the mistake of using sea salt containing dextrose, which is added as an anti-caking agent and is a form of sugar!

The chart on the next page shows the relative risk for cardiovascular events for different sodium intake levels. As you can see, the lowest point (lowest risk) is around 5 grams of sodium a day, which is about 2 teaspoons of sea salt (salt is about 40 percent sodium by weight). As much as 8 grams of sodium is still less risky than only 1 gram. This is why we recommend a daily goal of 4 to 6 grams of sodium, or about 2 to 2½ teaspoons of salt. This amount includes what you put on your food.

SODIUM LEVELS AND HAZARD RATIO OF CARDIOVASCULAR EVENTS[5]

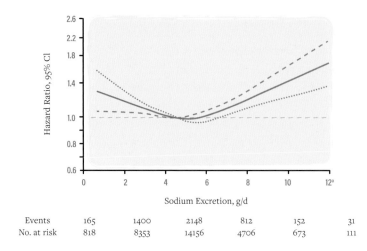

Events	165	1400	2148	812	152	31
No. at risk	818	8353	14156	4706	673	111

Potassium

If you don't want to lose muscle, pay attention here! Because you lose a lot of sodium through the diuretic effect (loss of water) of a low-carb diet, you will eventually lose a lot of potassium, too. Keeping your potassium level up safeguards your lean mass as you lose weight. Also, as with sodium, adequate potassium levels prevent cramping and fatigue. A deficiency in potassium causes low energy, heavy legs, salt cravings, dizziness, and heart flutter, and you might cry easily. Causes of low potassium can include dehydration from diarrhea, excessive sweating, and low-carb diets that are not well formulated.

Keeping up your sodium intake as well as your magnesium intake will help your body preserve potassium. Balancing your sodium and potassium intake is important as well. If you are getting 4 grams of sodium, you should be getting about 4.5 grams of potassium. For most people, 4 to 4.5 grams of sodium and 4.8 grams of potassium is a good target.

Your body needs 4.5 to 5 grams of potassium per day. To get an adequate amount, you can eat lots of foods that are high in potassium. A well-formulated ketogenic diet includes many sources of potassium. Here are some of them:

- **Animal proteins:** Beef, organ meats, pork, poultry, and seafood (Animal proteins are carb-free, too!)

POTASSIUM SUPPLEMENTS AND BLOOD PRESSURE MEDICATION

Do not take potassium supplements if you take blood pressure medication because the supplements can interfere with the medication. Check with your doctor before adding any potassium supplements.

BANANAS AND POTATOES AREN'T THE ONLY POTASSIUM SOURCES

I often teach nutrition classes. At the end of each class, I answer questions from the participants. One question I got was, "How do you recommend getting potassium if you don't recommend eating bananas or potatoes (especially if someone has high blood pressure)?"

I think it's interesting that doctors often recommend bananas and potatoes to their patients who have high blood pressure. Sure, these foods taste great, and people love them. In reality, though, those two foods are causing the problem; they're not going to fix it! Aside from that, there are foods that are much higher in potassium than the insulin-increasing banana and potato. Animal proteins contain almost as much, and in some cases more, potassium than bananas: 250 to 500 milligrams of potassium per 100 grams of animal protein versus 350 milligrams per 100 grams of banana. Dried herbs also have a lot more potassium without any of the sugar or starch. Avocados contain a lot of potassium, too.

Avocados

Dried herbs: Basil, chervil, dill, oregano, parsley, saffron, tarragon, and turmeric

Paprika and chili powder

If you need even more potassium than you can get from food, you can supplement with 99 milligrams of potassium twice daily.

Magnesium

Unlike a high-carb diet, a well-formulated ketogenic diet does not cause a massive depletion of magnesium in your body. For example, your body uses 54 milligrams of magnesium to process just 1 gram of sugar or starch, which creates a high demand for magnesium. No wonder magnesium deficiency is one of the most common deficiencies we see in our clients! About 70 percent of people don't even get the minimum recommended daily intake of magnesium. Most people who have metabolic syndrome or high blood pressure are magnesium deficient. Also, most people who are overweight, insulin resistant, or diabetic are deficient. Your insulin level increases as your blood pressure increases. Insulin stores magnesium, but if your insulin receptors are resistant and your cells grow resistant to insulin, you can't store magnesium; therefore, magnesium passes out of your body through urination.

Magnesium in your cells relaxes your muscles. If your magnesium level is too low, your blood vessels constrict rather than relax, which raises your blood pressure and decreases your energy level.

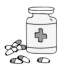

It is not entirely necessary to get a blood test to determine whether you are magnesium deficient because the fact is that most people don't get enough. We will always take magnesium supplements because it helps repair muscles, naturally relaxes blood vessels and tight muscles, and is a miracle cure for migraines and many other ailments. Good magnesium levels help regulate potassium levels. We also suggest giving children magnesium supplements because doing so can help with sleep issues. Babies can also benefit; supplemental magnesium helps them sleep better and stay calmer. In addition to magnesium tablets, you can get topical magnesium gels and lotions that are absorbed well.

You might be wondering why you need to supplement with minerals if our ancestors never did. Well, most of the magnesium they ingested was in the water they drank. Today, most people drink treated, softened, or bottled water, which is devoid of magnesium. Magnesium salts in water make deposits in water pipes and make it difficult to get soap to lather. These problems were solved with the development of water softeners and filtered city water, but the filtration process gets rid of the magnesium. Our ancestors drank untreated water from wells or streams that were rich in magnesium.

Because our water is now depleted of magnesium, and adequate amounts of magnesium aren't typically found in foods, we suggest taking 400 to 800 milligrams of a quality chelated magnesium supplement per day. Kids need an amount proportional to their weight: about 80 milligrams for one- to three-year-olds and about 130 milligrams for four- to eight-year-olds. Most of our clients and their children find magnesium relaxing, so they take it at bedtime to get quality sleep. In rare cases, magnesium is energizing rather than relaxing, so if you find yourself unable to sleep after taking it, we suggest taking 400 milligrams with breakfast and, if needed to manage muscle cramps or other symptoms, another 400-milligram dose at lunch. Everyone has a different tolerance to magnesium. The only problematic side effect is loose stools (something that happens when you take magnesium oxide, a non-absorbed form of magnesium). Always look for magnesium glycinate. If you are taking a small dose of magnesium glycinate and still have issues with loose stools, we suggest that you switch to a topical magnesium or use Epsom salts in the bath.

Two of the main symptoms of magnesium deficiency are hyperactivity and anxiety. In the standard American diet, a primary source of magnesium is fortified whole grains (which are grains to which a magnesium supplement has been added). So if you eliminate gluten from your diet, as we suggest, you are also eliminating a major source of magnesium. Because calcium competes with magnesium for uptake, taking calcium supplements without sufficient magnesium also increases the chance of magnesium deficiency.

Another thing to note when purchasing magnesium is that chelated magnesium is combined with an amino acid agent for absorption. If the dosage is 1,000 milligrams of magnesium citrate, the amount of magnesium isn't actually 1,000 milligrams. The chelated amino acid is heavier than magnesium, so about 15 percent of the weight is magnesium, and the rest is the amino acid agent. The only way to know how much magnesium you are getting is to look at the RDI (recommended daily intake). The RDI for magnesium is 400 milligrams per day. If a dose of the supplement delivers 50 percent of the RDI, then you know that each dose contains 200 milligrams of magnesium, regardless of what the dosage is on the front of the bottle.

Following are the different types of magnesium so you can choose the one that is best for you:

- **Magnesium citrate:** A mid-level form that will loosen stools.
- **Magnesium glycinate:** A calming and very absorbable form. Also helps lessen nerve pain.
- **Magnesium L-threonate:** An especially good form for brain function and cognition (for people with Alzheimer's disease and similar conditions).
- **Magnesium malate:** An energizing form that helps with cellular energy.
- **Magnesium oxide:** Not absorbable and will cause loose stools; a strong laxative.

NOTE

Having your blood tested for magnesium doesn't give you the whole picture. Blood levels of magnesium don't tell you what amount of magnesium is getting into your cells.

- **Magnesium orotate:** Helps supports heart health.
- **Magnesium sulfate** (also known as Epsom salts): Good for gastric issues or leaky gut syndrome when added to a cold foot soak at night. Also helps soothe sore muscles.
- **Magnesium taurate:** Helps support heart health and promotes calmness.

THE BENEFITS OF BEING KETO-ADAPTED

There are many benefits to being keto-adapted. Here are just a few you can expect:

- **Improved insulin sensitivity and recovery time between exercise sessions:** Being keto-adapted improves insulin sensitivity and speeds recovery time between training sessions. Well-formulated ketogenic diets are anti-inflammatory, which produces less oxidative stress during exercise, speeding recovery time between exercise sessions.
- **Muscle preservation:** Protein isn't oxidized, which preserves muscle. When you are a sugar burner, after you use up your glucose for fuel, your body steals from your muscle and bones to turn protein into more glucose. Branch chain amino acids (BCAA) are considered essential because your body can't make them, so you need to consume them for proper muscle building and repair (as well as replenishing red blood cells). We find it interesting that BCAA oxidation rates usually rise with exercise, which means you need more BCAA if you are an athlete. However, in keto-adapted athletes, ketones are burned in place of BCAA. Critics of low-carb diets claim that you need insulin to grow muscles. However, a well-designed low-carb, high-fat diet has less protein oxidation and double the amount of fat oxidation, which means your muscles are preserved while your body burns fat!
-  **Controlled pH and respiratory function:** The buildup of lactate is decreased, which helps control pH and respiratory function. A low-carb diet myth is that it puts you in a state of ketoacidosis. Often, doctors mistake nutritional ketosis

(blood ketones between 0.5 and 5.0 mmol) with ketoacidosis (blood ketones higher than 15 mmol). If you are in ketosis, your blood pH is healthy, and you don't have dips in pH because of lactate buildup and carbon dioxide during exercise (unlike a carb-consuming athlete).

- **Improved memory and cognition:** Ketones aren't just fuel for your body; they are also great for your brain. Ketones provide substrates (cholesterol) to help repair damaged neurons and membranes, which is why we push a high-fat, low-carb diet for clients who suffer from Alzheimer's disease (which researchers generally refer to as type 3 diabetes) and seizures. When the brain has become resistant to insulin, it has a hard time using glucose for fuel, but it can use ketones.

- **No immune system damage and less free radical damage:** When you are keto-adapted, your immune system isn't damaged, and there is less free radical damage in your cells. Free radicals are highly reactive molecules produced in the mitochondria that damage protein tissues and cell membranes. Free radicals develop as we exercise. However, ketones and free fatty acids are "clean-burning fuels." When the right kinds of fat (ketones or FFA) are the fuel source, reactive oxygen species (ROS or oxygen free radicals) are drastically reduced. Intense exercise on a high-carb diet overwhelms the antioxidant defenses and cell membranes, which explains why some extreme athletes have impaired immune systems and decreased gut (intestinal) health. A well-designed ketogenic diet not only fights off these aging antioxidants, but it also reduces inflammation of the gut, and it makes immune systems stronger than ever. We are no longer concerned about taking antioxidant supplements, and we don't worry about getting antioxidants from food (vegetables and especially fruit). As we show in Chapter 8, animal proteins are the real superfoods, and they don't come with inflammation-causing sugars.

PROTEIN-SPARING MODIFIED FASTING

As you become fully keto-adapted, eating less food becomes easier. Make sure that you keep your carb intake low and hit your protein goal, meaning less fat. So where's the limit?

In Chapter 9, we discuss water-only fasting, which has some good therapeutic benefits but can lead to a loss of lean mass (which is why it's important to eat well afterward). With this modified method of fasting, you reduce calories but maintain your valuable lean mass.

The idea behind a protein-sparing modified fast (PSMF) is to reduce carbs and fat as much as possible while still hitting your protein goal or even getting a bit more protein than your target. Instead of 0.8 times your lean mass for your protein goal, you want 1.0 times your lean mass when doing a PSMF. The additional protein makes your body use even more stored fat for fuel, helps break stalls or accelerate weight loss and healing, and helps keep you feeling full, while also giving you the added benefit of the high thermic effect of food with protein, which means that you effectively lose 25 percent of the calories you take.

You also want to get some fat during this type of fast to ensure that you keep your hormones happy and that fat-soluble vitamins (A, D, E, and K) get absorbed. Forty to 50 grams of fat will be enough.

PSMF is something we treat a bit like water fasting in that we suggest you do it every once in a while—maybe a day or two a week as needed to break a stall or increase weight loss.

For example, let's say a woman weighs 170 pounds and has 38 percent body fat, which means she has 105 pounds of lean mass. Her macros would be 20 grams or less of carbs, 105 grams of protein, and 40 grams of fat. As you can see, this is like fasting while preserving lean mass because she is only getting about 860 calories, though only about 730 of those calories are useful because of the thermic effect of food. She will get enough protein to preserve important lean body mass, but she will have to use a lot of stored fat to fuel her body. This is what makes PSMF such a great tool for accelerating weight loss or breaking a stall.

Pure Protein Day

In my first book, *Secrets to a Healthy Metabolism*, I wrote about what I call a "pure protein day." I knew there was a strong thermic effect of food with protein. My guideline for a pure protein day was no carbs (no vegetables, either) and little fat. I was afraid of the backlash from the keto community, so I started calling it a pure protein *and fat* day. However, now that Craig and I understand the science behind protein-sparing modified fasts, we know that the pure protein day works, and we were right all along! A pure protein day maintains muscle while you utilize the fat on your body to generate fuel and ketones. The thermic effect of the protein helps burn calories, too!

I often still eat my keto bread (I originally called it "protein bread") with scrambled eggs or a grass-fed beef burger.

Eight to ten years ago, Maria called this practice a "pure protein day." Back then, we hadn't heard of PSMF. We just knew the properties of the thermic effect of food and how our metabolisms worked, so we knew this could be helpful for people to lose weight faster. PSMF is becoming more popular and well-known and is a great tool for improving results.

KETO FAMILIES

A well-formulated ketogenic lifestyle has many benefits. However, there are other things that contribute to overall health and well-being. We see the keto lifestyle as a way to fix our diets, help our environment, change what we put on our skin, increase how we sleep, and much more.

The keto lifestyle is not only for adults who are trying to lose weight or heal; it can be wonderful for the whole family. We have worked with many families to help their kids improve their moods, behavior, focus, and so much more.

KETO FOR PREGNANCY AND INFANCY

Broken down by calories, the lean human body is 74 percent fat and 26 percent protein. Fat is a structural part of every human cell and is the preferred fuel source of the mitochondria, which are the energy-burning units of each cell. A fetus naturally uses ketones before and immediately after birth. Many studies done on pregnant

My daughter (11 years old) was told she was borderline insulin resistant and that she had ADHD and a behavior disorder. [On keto] she has lost 38 pounds and no longer has any symptoms of any of her conditions. She sleeps better at night and has amazing grades in school this year, her first year in junior high.

pigs that are placed on ketogenic diets show fetuses with increased fetal brain weight, cell size, and protein content.

In the early stages of pregnancy, there is an upsurge in body fat accumulation, which is connected to hyperphagia and increased lipogenesis. In the later stages of pregnancy, there is an accelerated breakdown of fat depots, which plays an important role in fetal development.

The fetus uses fatty acids from the placenta as well as two other products: glycerol and ketone bodies. Even though glycerol goes through the placenta in small proportions, it is a superior substrate for "maternal gluconeogenesis." Heightened ketogenesis in fasting conditions—or with the addition of MCT oils—creates an easy transference of ketones to the fetus. This transfer allows maternal ketone bodies to reach the fetus, where the ketones can be used as fuels for oxidative metabolism as well as lipogenic substrates.

The fat-soluble vitamins A, D, E, and K are essential for the formation of healthy fetuses. Full-fat dairy is also filled with healthy cholesterol, but some people are dairy-sensitive. For those particular clients, we suggest finding other sources of saturated fats, such as coconut oil and quality animal fats, seafood, and egg yolks.

We all know that breast milk is the healthiest thing for a baby. Breast milk is naturally very high in fat—more than 60 percent fat; it's loaded with both saturated fat and cholesterol. The macros in breast milk are specifically designed to meet babies' needs for growing their brains and bodies. If a newborn is breastfed, the baby is always in ketosis, and ketosis helps develop and build babies' brains. Keto-adapted babies can efficiently turn ketone bodies into acetyl-CoA and myelin. Those needs don't change suddenly when babies move into early childhood and are no longer breastfed.

KETO KIDS

This lifestyle can have amazing results for kids, too. We all want our kids to grow up and have a happy, healthy life, and good nutrition starts in childhood. Let's take a look at what happens when kids get too much sugar in their diets and what happens when they eat too many carbohydrates.

No matter where the carbohydrates are being stored—the liver or the muscles—the body's total storage capacity for carbohydrates is quite limited. Once stored, the body must use the rest of the fuel or convert it to triglycerides to be stored as fat. As we discuss in Chapter 3, oxidative priority dictates that all the fat that was eaten with those carbs gets directly stored in the fat cells while the body deals with the high glucose levels caused by the excess carbohydrates that have been eaten. However, that's not the worst of it. Any meal or snack that is high in carbohydrates generates a rapid rise in blood glucose.

The pancreas secretes the hormone insulin to adjust for this rapid rise in glucose. Insulin then lowers the levels of blood glucose. However, the pancreas overcorrects when there is a very high load of carbohydrates, which causes your blood sugar to drop; usually about two hours after eating, you are hungry again due to low blood glucose. Cravings, usually for sweets, are frequently part of this cycle, and those cravings lead you to snack on more carbohydrates. Not eating makes you feel ravenous, shaky, moody, and ready to "crash." This cycle keeps insulin elevated and causes you never to rid yourself of that extra stored fat.

High insulin levels also suppress two important hormones: growth hormone and glucagon. Growth hormone is used for muscle development and building new muscle mass. Glucagon promotes the burning of fat and sugar.

This type of high sugar diet can also lead to a lot of mood issues, ADHD, problems focusing, and lots of other conditions that can hold your kid back.

We are seeing more and more cases of diabetes in children. It is the same process of developing overstuffed and inflamed fat cells as adults, just massively accelerated to only a few years of life.

A STICK IN THE MUD?

I received a comment on Facebook saying that I am a "stick-in-the-mud mom" because I don't let my boys eat at frozen yogurt shops. At first, that comment hurt, but then I realized that my kids are lucky because they enjoy tasty treats made with love while we are out exploring nature and riding bikes rather than sitting in an air-conditioned, fluorescent-lit ice cream shop! I know that someday my boys will appreciate all the time I put into making quality, tasty, and healthy food for them!

KETO IS GREAT FOR CHILDREN, TOO

Our sons eat roughly the same way we do, and they are thriving. When they came home with us at ages one and two, they barely registered on the height and weight charts. We immediately started feeding them the foods we ate (including bone broth for Kai). Now, they are six and seven years old, and they are at the seventy-fifth percentile on the height and weight charts.

A lifestyle like this not only reverses the damage caused by years of high-sugar and high-carb eating, it can protect our kids from suffering metabolic issues later in life.

Our kids deserve to feel their best and have the mental clarity, focus, improved moods, and more that come with being keto-adapted. Also, later in life, they will have more energy for sports, less acne, and more focus. Keto is a wonderful lifestyle for the whole family.

MODIFICATIONS FOR KIDS

There are two modifications we make for kids who are still growing:

- We don't have our children do any intermittent fasting. They eat three meals a day and maybe have an evening snack. However, the diet we recommend is still much different from the diet of a typical child who snacks all day long. For the most part, our boys fill up at each meal and have little to no snacks in between.

REFINED SUGARS ARE TOXIC

Our boys never eat refined sugar. Once, on an airplane, we asked the flight attendant for a sugar-free drink for Kai. She mistakenly brought him juice containing lots of sugar. After drinking just one serving, he threw up. The moral? Refined sugar is toxic to our bodies. We are always careful to pack the boys' lunches when they go to camp, and we homeschool them due in part to all the junk food they would be bombarded with at public schools.

- We don't limit their protein. Whereas an adult will have a protein goal of 0.8 times their lean body mass, kids can eat two or even three times their lean mass in protein each day. Our boys each weigh about 50 pounds, but they easily get 100 grams or more of protein a day; some days, it is closer to 150 grams. Protein is what helps kids grow, so don't limit their protein intake, and let them eat the fats that come with that protein. Carbohydrates, however, have nothing to do with growth. As we discuss in Chapter 8, animal proteins are some of the most nutrient-dense foods out there. Along with the protein, they will be getting tons of nutrients to help their growing bodies and brains thrive.

Don't be afraid to bring the whole family along when following the ketogenic lifestyle. They will be better for it, and your life will be easier because everyone can eat the same meals!

AN IDEAL KETO DAY FOR HEALING AND WEIGHT LOSS

 ## MORNING

- Wake up with the sun, and if you can, go outside and expose as much skin to the sun as possible for twenty minutes within the first two hours of waking. Doing so starts your circadian clock.

- Drink ice-cold water instead of hot coffee; cold water shrinks mitochondria, making them more efficient. Plus, good water (no chlorine or fluoride) is essential for cellular health.

- Work out if possible, because exercise builds healthy mitochondria. The best way to burn fat is to perform aerobic exercise first thing in the morning on an empty stomach. To avoid dehydration, drink a large glass of water. You burn 300 percent more body fat in the morning on an empty stomach than at any other time in the day because your body does not have any glycogen or stored carbohydrates/sugar in the liver to burn. When this happens, your body must go directly into the fat stores to get the energy necessary to complete the activity. You also increase the level of human growth hormone, which is the fat-burning hormone. The human growth hormone and insulin counteract each other. If one is high, the other is low, like a see-saw. If you eat before a workout—particularly carbohydrates—your insulin levels will spike, meaning your growth hormone levels will be low. If possible, exercise outside. Get sunlight! Even in below-zero weather, we run outside. Those cold morning runs have many benefits:
  - Being outside in nature.
  - Getting sunlight.
  - Getting cold therapy, which has many health benefits. For more on cold therapy, see Chapter 12.
  - Exercising (despite the temperature) to build healthy mitochondria.

- Try to take an ice-cold shower (or as cold as you can stand). At a minimum, make the shower as cold as you can handle for the last few minutes. Cold therapy like this helps improve mitochondrial efficiency, increases the amount of brown fat, and speeds recovery. Read more about cold therapy in Chapter 12.

MIDDAY

- Break your fast with a ketogenic meal.
- Wear grounding shoes or walk barefoot. Place a grounding mat under your desk to make your cells more alkaline or negatively charged. Read more about grounding in Chapter 12.
- Drink lots of water.

EVENING

- Limit exposure to blue light:
  - Set electronics to lower blue light (use the Night Shift setting on iOS devices).
  - Wear blue-blocking glasses when watching TV or working on a computer.
- Dunk your face in ice water or jump into ice-cold water. (Maria swims in a spring-fed river before bedtime.) Cold therapy before bed can help with sleep. Read more about cold therapy in Chapter 12.
- To lower your body temperature, have a keto snow cone—shaved ice with natural sugar-free flavorings. (We love Everly water enhancers.)
- Limit vigorous exercise. Stick to gentle walking or yoga in the evening.

BEDTIME

- Do not eat within three hours of bedtime.
- Keep your bedroom cooler than 68°F; the lower the temperature, the better. We also have a cooling mattress pad (a ChiliPad).
- Use light-blocking blinds to keep your bedroom dark.
- Use a sound machine to add sound to the bedroom to help with sleep.
- Use an essential oil diffuser to emit a lavender scent.
- Sleep eight to ten hours every night!

This is an example of an ideal day for healing and weight loss. It can also be ideal for maintenance, although a maintenance day would include more calories (fat) during the eating window.

Dive in and give it a try. You will be amazed at how good your body can feel and how much energy you have. You'll also notice improved moods, mental clarity, and focus. Make food and your environment your medicine for better health!

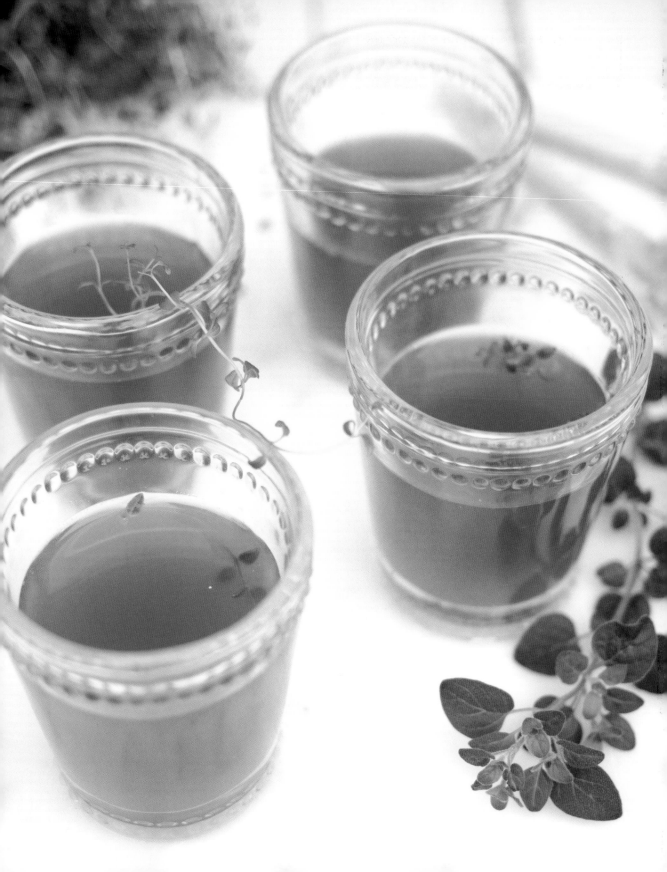

chapter 5

Hormones

A ketogenic diet allows you to manage your hormones by creating a negative fat flux (increased lipolysis; see Chapter 3). Hormones play a big role in how you feel, your hunger, your moods, your food cravings, and much more.

The first thing a ketogenic diet does is stabilize your insulin levels and restore leptin signaling. Having less insulin around means that you will feel full longer and have fewer food cravings. When your insulin spikes because of a high carb intake, your insulin level always overcorrects, meaning that it goes from being really high to being really low. These fluctuations in insulin cause hunger and energy crashes; as a result, you feel as though you need to eat every two hours. Eating keto also restores leptin signaling and helps you feel the "I'm full" signal.

This chapter introduces you to the different hormones and the roles each one plays in the body.

HORMONES RUN OUR METABOLISMS

When we start talking about hormones and weight, clients usually get a surprised look on their faces. Hormones are

- Chemical messengers from cells in the body
- Produced by almost every organ system
- Secreted directly into the bloodstream

Hormones signal certain cells to perform certain functions. Hormones are in charge of many important pieces of our everyday lives, including mood swings, sex drive, blood sugar levels, muscle tone, fat-burning ability, metabolism, and the immune system. The list is huge! Hormones play a role in everything from good sleep and good sex to headaches, stress, fatigue, and weight gain.

Losing weight can be a struggle, and many people believe that there must be a reason the weight is not coming off. It is true that hormonal imbalance affects some overweight individuals. Hormones do play a role in weight loss and weight gain, but the role is dependent on the individual and his or her dietary and exercise habits.

Hormones can affect our moods and energy levels. Our way of life plays a huge role in our hormonal makeup. For example, if a person is inactive, certain hormones, such as testosterone, decrease. Testosterone is a hormone that works to increase metabolism, which means it plays a role in regulating weight and encouraging weight loss. In addition, a more active person has a greater number of healthy mitochondria, the power centers of our cells, which helps enhance hormone balance. Hormone balance is essential so the body can cope with its own need to adapt to stress during physical exertion. As a result, the body creates balanced hormones, which boost metabolism and lead to weight loss. By exercising regularly, getting adequate sleep, and eating the right foods (and avoiding the foods that can mess with hormone balance), your body can create harmony with your hormones.

THE THYROID GLAND

We like to compare the thyroid gland to the cruise control system in a car. Cruise control keeps the car running at a constant speed without the driver having to keep a steady foot on the gas pedal. The hormone produced by the thyroid does the same thing: It keeps part of the body working at the proper speed. However, problems arise if the thyroid starts to malfunction. Two common thyroid conditions are hypothyroidism and hyperthyroidism:

- **Hypothyroidism:** If thyroid hormone levels decrease—a condition known as hypothyroidism—the rest of your body processes decrease in activity, which means that the cells need less energy (calories) and extra energy is stored as fat. Weight increases even though the appetite decreases. Often, a person with hypothyroidism feels cold because the body is producing less heat and the sweat glands no longer keep the skin moist. The brain wants to sleep all the time, the heart beats slower, the basal metabolic rate slows, and the bowels become sluggish. The whole body slows down.

- **Hyperthyroidism:** If thyroid levels increase—a condition known as hyperthyroidism—other body processes increase activity, which means more energy (calories) is used. Fat and protein stores are mobilized and weight decreases even as appetite increases. Patients with hyperthyroidism often feel hot because the body produces more heat and sweating increases to cool down. The brain is working overtime, which causes irritability and shakiness. Sleep becomes difficult, which makes symptoms worse. The heartbeat speeds up and bowel activity increases. The whole body speeds up, and cells age at a faster rate.

The thyroid has profound effects on our metabolism, fertility, growth, and development, as well as our cardiovascular and central nervous systems.

- **Metabolism:** Thyroid hormones fuel complex metabolic activities that increase your basal metabolic rate. The thyroid can cause an increase in body heat production, which increases oxygen consumption and the rate at which ATP (adenosine triphosphate, our cellular energy source) is released. There are two types of metabolism:

  1. **Fat metabolism:** Increased thyroid hormone levels boost fat mobilization; this amplifies concentrations of fatty acids in your blood. Blood concentrations of cholesterol and triglycerides are inversely connected with thyroid hormone levels, which means that as thyroid hormone levels go up, concentrations of cholesterol and triglycerides go down (and vice versa). For example, hypothyroidism is linked to high blood cholesterol levels.

  2. **Carbohydrate metabolism:** Thyroid hormones fuel our bodies' ability to burn carbohydrates. Hypothyroidism can increase the risk of diabetes because our thyroid enhances insulin-dependent entry of glucose into cells to generate free glucose.

- **Fertility:** Thyroid hormones control our sex hormones. Hypothyroidism is frequently associated with infertility.

- **Growth:** Thyroid hormones are necessary for normal growth. Thyroid deficiencies in children result in growth retardation. The human growth hormone and the thyroid hormones are intimately connected.

- **Development:** An experiment on tadpoles demonstrated the effects of the thyroid on development. The tadpoles were deprived of thyroid hormones, which resulted in an inability to endure metamorphosis into frogs. Thyroid hormones are vital for fetal brain development, which is one reason why adequate iodine is important for brain development in children. Iodine helps make healthy thyroid hormones.

- **Cardiovascular system:** Thyroid hormones control heart rate, contractility, and cardiac output. The thyroid's hormones also support blood flow to many organs.

- **Central nervous system:** Thyroid hormones control your mental state. Hypothyroid patients often feel mentally sluggish, whereas hyperthyroid patients often feel anxious and irritable.[1]

REGULATING THYROID OUTPUT

The thyroid runs many parts of the body. Making a few diet and lifestyle changes can help regulate your thyroid output. Some foods, such as cruciferous veggies, can aggravate existing thyroid issues because they contain enzymes that interfere with thyroid output. Sleep and exercise—specifically yoga—can be very therapeutic for the thyroid.

Follow these steps for success:

- **Cut all chlorine and fluoride out of your diet.** Both are often found in unfiltered water supplies. Reverse-osmosis filtered water is a better alternative. Chlorine and fluoride—even from swimming or soaking in chlorinated water—wreak havoc on your thyroid.

- **Get your iodine on!** Low iodine levels cause poor thyroid function, leading to miscarriages, poor brain development in babies and children, constipation, and poor circulation. Sea salt is devoid of iodine, so you need to get iodine from other sources. Eggs, seafood (including oysters, scallops, and shrimp), and fish (especially cod, salmon, tuna, and sardines) are good sources of iodine.

- **Take amino acids.** Your thyroid demands amino acids, which are found in animal proteins. Amino acids, such as L-tyrosine, are necessary for the synthesis of thyroid hormone and cortisol. L-tyrosine is found in red meat and other animal proteins. Tyrosine can also be made by another amino acid, phenylalanine, but phenylalanine needs iron for conversion. Many women lack iron and end up with low thyroid function.

- **Get adequate zinc.** The thyroid is a zinc hog! You lose a lot of zinc as you sweat, and a zinc deficiency is often a cause of acne or "backne" (acne on the back), hypothyroidism, and depressed immune function. Red meat, oysters, crab, lobster, and chicken are great sources of zinc.

- **Take selenium.** Optimally, you need 200 micrograms each day; selenium is essential for the conversion of T4 to T3, the active form of thyroid hormone. You can get this amount simply by eating two Brazil nuts a day. Yellowfin tuna, halibut, sardines, and grass-fed beef are also good sources of selenium. Alternatively, you can get an adequate amount of selenium by taking supplements.

- **Avoid fructose.** Although fructose doesn't raise blood sugar like other forms of sugar, it is metabolized in the liver. Over time, this leads to a buildup of fat in the liver. T4 is converted to the activated thyroid hormone T3 in the liver rather than in the thyroid. A fatty liver has a harder time converting T4 to activated T3. For more liver cleansing tips, see page 294.

Take Selenium While Pregnant

During pregnancy, a woman's immune system goes into overdrive to protect the fetus. Once the baby is born, the woman develops antibodies against her thyroid. Taking 200 micrograms of selenium while pregnant is very safe for both mother and fetus and is helpful for lowering the autoimmune response after birth.

THE GLUCAGON-INSULIN CONNECTION

We'd like to introduce you to an awesome fat-burning hormone called glucagon. Don't confuse glucagon with glycogen, however:

- **Glucagon** is the opposite hormone to insulin.
- **Glycogen** is stored sugar in the muscles and liver that increases insulin.

Insulin takes the sugars and carbohydrates you eat and stores them as fat or glycogen. Glucagon takes that stored glycogen and tells the liver to turn it into glucose in the blood. When stored glycogen is depleted, glucagon tells the liver to turn protein (amino acids from lean mass) into glucose via gluconeogenesis. Glucagon goes up when blood sugar dips, meaning that it is a demand-driven process.

In the presence of insulin, you can't burn fat for energy. Lipolysis is stopped when insulin is raised. Eating the typical American diet of sugar, refined carbohydrates, and fat-free foods stops fat burning. Overconsumption of any food increases insulin and stops lipolysis (and lowers glucagon). Not only does this prevent fat burning, but it also activates the storage of fat by making triglycerides to store in adipose tissue (fat cells).

Glucagon is also stimulated by exercise; exercise increases glucagon by up to five times our normal levels! If you combine exercise and increased amounts of protein, you can strategically enhance weight loss. Exercise also decreases insulin levels.

Initially, low-calorie diets increase glucagon, too, which is why people lose some weight by not eating or by fasting.

Follow these steps to increase glucagon:

- Eat adequate amounts of protein.
- Keep your liver healthy. Cut all alcohol and high-carb foods that cause fatty liver.
- Exercise!

HUMAN GROWTH HORMONE (HGH)

Human growth hormone (HGH) is an amazing hormone that is produced by the pituitary gland in the brain. This hormone stimulates cell production and is responsible for increasing height, building muscle mass, keeping bones healthy, controlling sugar and insulin levels, absorbing calcium, as well as helping numerous other functions that are fundamental for growth. However, we don't recommend supplementing with HGH because it can come with some scary side effects. You can boost this hormone naturally through diet and exercise.

HGH is produced at full speed when we are young, but production slows as we age. HGH levels peak during puberty, when there is a growth spurt, and continue to decline throughout adulthood, especially after age 30. This decrease in HGH is what causes a loss of skin elasticity (wrinkles), increased issues with diabetes, depression, loss of energy, and loss of muscle mass. Increasing the levels of HGH can make you look young and feel healthy.

Diet, exercise, and sleep patterns all play roles in human growth hormone secretion. This hormone regulates a lot of important physiological functions, including water and energy balance, reproductive activity, and the activity of other glands. HGH is also involved in important processes that control metabolism, including regulating muscle, bone, and collagen, regulating fat burning, and preserving a healthy body composition. There is no doubt that increasing the secretion of natural HGH is favorable to everyone, including those with joint pain, diabetes, blood sugar imbalances, arthritis, abnormal heart growth, muscle weakness, and increased triglycerides.

It has recently been discovered that people can have a growth hormone deficiency, which proves just how important this hormone is. People with a deficiency have a considerably low muscle mass and high body fat; most were obese, had an increased risk of heart disease, and a reduced ability to exercise.

The release of human growth hormone can be triggered by some natural stimuli, the most powerful of which are sleep and exercise. In healthy bodies, human growth hormone secretion follows a circadian rhythm and is released in six to twelve distinct portions per day, with the largest portion secreted about an hour after the onset of nighttime sleep. Because the largest portion of HGH is secreted while you are sleeping, we stress the importance of sleep!

It is imperative for everyone—athletes most of all— to get plenty of sleep. Most Olympic athletes get about ten hours of sleep each night. We make sure to get ten hours of sleep, too! If the quality of sleep is insufficient, there will be a decline in the amount of human growth hormone released, with negative consequences for our overall physical and mental health. Significant prerequisites for good quality sleep and optimal HGH secretion during sleep include a cool, dark room and a quality diet containing sufficient protein (for more information, see Chapter 12). Sleep is necessary for good health in general, and for most people, this means around eight hours.

Specific exercise routines and nutritional strategies can enhance the natural secretion of HGH. There is no need to inject dangerous, unnatural hormones to achieve higher levels; you just need to work to stimulate secretion in a safe way. Various studies find that HGH is triggered by exercise-induced increases in adrenaline, nitric oxide, lactate, and nerve activity. To achieve a surge of HGH with exercise, you need to spend at least ten minutes working above lactate threshold intensity, which means you will be sweating and feeling the "burn."[2] A major surge of HGH will occur, with levels declining gradually over a period of an hour.

 Multiple daily workouts can give a boost to optimal HGH secretion over a twenty-four-hour period. That is why we suggest breaking up your exercise into two smaller, yet harder, workout times throughout your day.

As far as diet is concerned, athletes are normally pushed to eat a diet high in carbohydrates, consuming foods with a higher glycemic index around intense exercise and consuming starchy carbohydrates at other times of the day. The standard advice with regard to fluids is to drink carbohydrate-electrolyte drinks before, during, and after exercise.

However, high-carb diets switch off HGH secretion, and carb-loading after exercise is not a good strategy for increasing the secretion of HGH. Foods high in carbohydrates stimulate insulin release, which, in turn, contributes to a reduction in HGH. American athletes are the only athletes who encourage the "carb loading" theory. The 2008 Kenyan Olympic marathon winner Samuel Wanjiru ate a huge steak with broccoli for his pre-race meal—not a plate of pasta. (And his lips have never touched a bottle of Gatorade!) More and more athletes are following a ketogenic diet for better performance and quicker recovery times.

Hydration is also a huge piece of keeping that HGH firing. Drinking plenty of water with electrolytes during exercise is extremely important because dehydration has been found to reduce the exercise-induced HGH response drastically.

HGH is responsible for our youthful physique and well-being. Natural methods of enhancing this hormone can reap a multitude of benefits. Sticking with keto foods and muscle-stimulating exercise is a safe and effective way to increase this hormone.

Use these tips for successfully increasing your HGH levels:

- Stay hydrated. Keep water and electrolytes (sodium, potassium, and magnesium) up.

- Perform muscle-stimulating exercise a few times a week.

- Break exercise into two shorter workouts rather than one long one.
- Get at least eight hours of quality sleep every night.
- Do not eat three hours before bed. The largest surge of HGH occurs thirty minutes after you fall asleep, but its antagonist is insulin. If you eat before bed, you will not benefit from this surge of your fat-burning hormone.
- Do not eat before exercising. Human growth hormone and insulin counteract each other. Like a seesaw, if one is high, the other is low. If you eat before a workout—especially carbohydrates—your insulin levels will spike, meaning your growth hormone levels will be low.

LEPTIN

Have you ever wondered why it is easier to gain weight than to keep it off? The key is in the fat cells, where the powerful hormone leptin is produced. Leptin signals the brain to regulate the metabolism to store or to burn fat.

Research shows that an estimate of more than 85 percent of the people who lose weight end up regaining it because the body's "metabolic thermostat"—leptin—is reset upward automatically.[3] When people lose weight, leptin production decreases, which causes people to regain the lost weight. This protein-bound hormone is derived from fat cells, so when you lose fat, leptin levels drop. When you gain fat, leptin levels rise. After leptin is secreted by your fat cells, it travels to the hypothalamus, which controls eating behavior. Once leptin reaches the hypothalamus, it activates anorectic nerve cells, which decreases your appetite. At the same time, leptin stops cells from stimulating your appetite. To put it simply, when leptin levels drop, you get hungry. When they go up, you feel full.

As well as being affected by total body fat levels, leptin levels rise and fall quite rapidly in response to both overfeeding and underfeeding. After the initial drop in response to underfeeding, leptin declines at a rate that's linked more closely to the loss of fat.

Some scientists refer to leptin as an "anti-obesity hormone," but it is now being called an "anti-starvation" hormone because it tells our brains what to do when our fat stores are in short supply.

To demonstrate the power of leptin, scientists gave leptin injections to lean volunteers and obese volunteers who had recently lost weight. The team found that most of the metabolic and hormonal changes were reversed once leptin levels were restored to pre-weight-loss levels, which means the volunteers had a hard time keeping the weight from creeping back on. In the study, subjects were fed 800 calories per day until they'd lost 10 percent of their weight.[4] The 800-calorie diet led to a drop in both leptin and thyroid hormone concentrations, along with a reduction in the metabolic rate. For the next five weeks, the subjects were given low-dose leptin injections twice a day to bring leptin back to pre-diet levels. These injections of leptin reversed the drop in energy expenditure and increased thyroid hormone levels. The participants also continued to lose fat while preserving muscle tissue.

Another impact is that a drop in leptin concentrations seems to play a larger effect on your body than increasing leptin levels above the normal physiological range. The primary functional role of leptin is to defend, rather than reduce, body fat by increasing appetite and decreasing energy expenditure when fat stores are low. Physiological responses to levels of leptin below and above this threshold are very unbalanced. Low levels of leptin trigger a strong counter-regulation to a "perceived" threat to survival.[5] Your body has to fight harder against losing fat than it does against gaining fat. That's why most people find it a whole lot easier to get fat than they do to get lean.

Unfortunately, there is no easy route of just taking a leptin pill to help solve our weight problems. First, leptin can't be taken orally because our stomach can't absorb it. Leptin needs to be injected for it to be absorbed, which is both inconvenient and very expensive.

A more practical and healthy solution is to follow a diet of cycling your calorie and fat intake throughout the course of a week. A day of controlled overeating (additional fat and protein) raises leptin levels and can help you avoid some of the metabolic adaptations that naturally occur with any restricted-calorie diet. We aren't talking about a full-blown "cheat day"—not like you might be thinking, anyway. Full-blown "cheat days" can undo all the hard work you've done during the previous six days.

Instead, people who are restricting calories can profit from a kind of planned break during the week. Having a higher-calorie day during the week can help with leptin. Mixing this with a protein-sparing modified fast day (see page 88) once or twice a week can be a good combination for shaking up the metabolic set point and increasing leptin sensitivity.

LEPTIN RESISTANCE

After all this information, you might think that having extra fat stores creates more leptin. However, that is where an interesting mystery comes into play because the majority of those who are significantly overweight are also leptin resistant. Most defects in leptin signaling may lead to obesity, overeating, and less energy expenditure. Leptin resistance occurs after being overexposed to high levels of the hormone. At this point, the body no longer responds to the leptin, which can result in the development of leptin resistance.

The best way to reduce your chances of diabetes is to avoid surges in leptin, which is the leading cause of leptin resistance. Eating the typical American diet, full of refined sugars and other processed foods, is a guaranteed way to cause undesired surges. Focusing on nutrient-dense, unprocessed whole foods, like animal proteins, is the best way to prevent leptin resistance.

To recap: After you eat, your body releases leptin, which tells your body to stop feeling hungry and to start burning calories. An interesting paradox is that the more fat your body carries, the more leptin you produce. However, your body starts to become resistant in a way that is like insulin resistance. The objective is to optimize your levels of this hormone by eating foods that increase your body's sensitivity to leptin and eating foods that work with other hormones to regulate leptin's functions.

Very nutrient-dense, quality animal proteins can improve leptin sensitivity—especially those high in omega-3s (such as fish). EPA is especially good at stimulating leptin, so get foods high in EPA such as salmon, mackerel, sardines, and herring. Zinc also increases leptin, so eating oysters is a great option. Red meat, seafood, and chicken also are high in zinc.

Follow these tips for successfully combating leptin resistance:

- Once a week, overfeed yourself (eat 400 to 600 calories of added fat and protein, not added carbs).
- Eat foods high in omega-3 fats.
- Eat foods high in zinc.

GHRELIN

Scientists believe they have discovered why people get hungry at mealtimes, why dieters who lose weight often gain it back, and why stomach surgery helps obese people lose a great deal of weight. One main reason is a hormone called ghrelin, which makes us hungry, slows metabolism, and decreases the body's ability to burn fat.

Ghrelin creates ravenous cravings for food. Even simple food habits can increase ghrelin. Our bodies increase the production of this hormone before eating, and it can be triggered by different factors—whether it is the clock striking noon or the delicious smells wafting out of a bakery as you walk by.

Ghrelin levels increase before meals and drop afterward. Volunteers given ghrelin injections felt extremely hungry, and, when turned loose at a buffet, ate 30 percent more than they did previously.[6] Dieters who lose weight produce more ghrelin than they did before dieting as if their bodies are fighting against starvation. By contrast, obese people who have gastric bypass surgery to lose weight end up with low levels of ghrelin, which helps explain why their appetites decrease noticeably after the surgery. Your stomach is like a rubber band; you can stretch it out when you eat a lot. When you constantly stretch this rubber band,

REPLACING BAD HABITS WITH GOOD ONES

I grew up on a bedtime snack, and that snack was often junk food, such as toast with peanut butter and honey or ice cream sandwiches. For eighteen years I ate a snack before bed. It was the hardest habit for me to break because, even though I wasn't actually hungry, my ghrelin increased when the clock struck 8:30 p.m.; that was the time my brain told me to eat. I had to replace that bad habit with a healthy one. It was extremely difficult, but I had to distract my belly from believing it was time for food. I started practicing yoga instead, and that switch helped me reverse this poor eating routine.

causing it to be always extended, it eventually stays a larger size. Having an extended stomach causes you to produce more ghrelin and to be hungry, which causes a snowball effect of weight gain and constant hunger. This is in part due to calorie-rich but nutrient-deficient foods, like sugar and processed foods. You can eat large volumes of these foods and still not get the nutrients your body needs. By not overconsuming food, you are in control of shrinking your rubber band, which helps with managing ghrelin.

Another factor in ghrelin production is the amount of sleep you get. People who fail to sleep properly overstimulate their ghrelin production, which increases the desire for food. Getting the right amount of sleep (eight hours or more) can be the first step to making sure that you're getting the ghrelin and leptin balance that your body needs to maintain a healthy weight naturally. Remember that you can't make up for lost sleep on the weekends; you have to try to get a consistent amount of sleep each night.

Also, we say that you need to get "quality" sleep because many people suffer from sleep apnea and don't know it. If you have been told you snore, kick, talk, or stop breathing in the night, have your doctor check for sleep apnea. Sleep disorders will keep you from getting into REM sleep, which is when our hormones are balanced.

Another factor in the suppression of ghrelin production is the amount of protein you eat and how much hydrochloric acid you produce. If you have a slow thyroid, you often lack sufficient hydrochloric acid, which increases hunger and lack of satisfaction because your cells are still hungry. You are not able to absorb nutrients without adequate amounts of hydrochloric acid. You also slowly lower production of hydrochloric acid as you age. Getting enough protein for the day and having sufficient hydrochloric acid is very important for managing ghrelin levels.

A LACK OF SLEEP OVERSTIMULATES GHRELIN PRODUCTION

If I get a poor night of sleep or stay up late for a wedding or get-together, I notice that I'm extra hungry the next day. I still always wake up early, and I feel like I have endless hunger all day. In addition to overstimulating ghrelin, lack of sleep reduces the production of leptin, which is the body's appetite suppressant. In short, if you don't get enough sleep, the hormones in your body get all out of whack, and you think that you're hungry when you don't really need to eat.

Scientists have created an anti-obesity vaccine that reduces the production of ghrelin, which helps reduce cravings. Yes, these drugs are on the market, but instead of putting a huge dent in your wallet, you can start to balance ghrelin by following a few easy steps. Use these guidelines for successfully maintaining proper ghrelin levels:

- Get adequate sleep without prescription sleep medications.
- Change bad habits, such as eating at bedtime, to change your brain signals.
- Eat adequate protein to manage ghrelin hormones.
- Do not overstretch your stomach with large volumes of food. Eat nutrient-dense foods like animal proteins.
- If you have a slow thyroid or lack of hydrochloric acid, supplement with 500 to 700 milligrams of HCl with pepsin before meals. You could be eating nutrient-dense foods, but if you don't have enough hydrochloric acid, you won't benefit from the added nutrients because your body won't be able to utilize them.
- Treat your hunger like a muscle. You need to flex it to build its strength.

OBESITY AND SLEEP APNEA

You don't have to be overweight to suffer from sleep apnea. For example, did you know that allergies are a primary cause of sleep apnea? Often, we think apnea is a side effect of obesity, but now we are learning that apnea actually often causes obesity—not the other way around! Sleep apnea causes issues with hormones, such as ghrelin, which causes a lack of feeling full, resulting in overeating and weight gain. Too often, we blame ourselves for lack of control with food; however, hormones are extremely powerful messengers that take control of you! Getting down to the root cause of overeating (such as a hormone imbalance) is the only way to deal with the problem. Our traditional medical professionals have been failing us, such as by throwing prescriptions for sleep medications at patients who don't sleep well. Unfortunately, those prescriptions often cause weight gain and damage the mitochondria.

ESTROGEN AND PROGESTERONE

Estrogen and progesterone are powerful hormones that balance our moods, temperature, menstrual cycle, cravings, fat burning, fat storage, and much more. Female hormone-related problems are on the rise. About 60 percent of women suffer from PMS. Also, women suffer from an excess of hormonal imbalance symptoms, some menopausal and others not. There is strong evidence that the proper hormonal balance necessary for a woman's body to function healthily is being interfered with by several factors, including nutrition.

Research has shown that many women in their thirties, and some even younger than that, will sporadically not ovulate. Without ovulation, maturation of a woman's follicles doesn't occur, and no progesterone is made. A progesterone deficiency occurs, and several problems can result, including the month-long occurrence of unopposed estrogen, which comes with lots of side effects.

A second major problem resulting from the imbalance is the link between progesterone loss and stress. Stress in combination with a bad diet can provoke cycles in which ovulation does not occur. The consequent lack of progesterone slows the production of the stress-busting hormones, aggravating stressful conditions that give rise to further anovulatory months, and so continues the unhealthy cycle.

A new scientific discovery now links a surprising factor to this estrogen and progesterone imbalance. The industrialized world we now live in is filled with something called petrochemical derivatives. They are in the air, food, and water. They include pesticides and herbicides, such as DDT; they're also in various plastics found in baby bottles and water jugs, as well as in PCBs (polychlorinated biphenyl). These chemicals mimic estrogen and are highly fat-soluble. They are not biodegradable and are not well excreted from our bodies, and they gather in our fat tissues. These chemicals have a mysterious ability to mimic natural estrogen and therefore are called xenoestrogens. Even though they are foreign chemicals, they are gathered up by the estrogen receptor sites in our bodies, seriously interfering with natural biochemical activity. Drinking sodas out of plastic bottles is one of the leading causes of estrogen dominance.

Extensive research is now revealing an alarming situation worldwide: Too much bad estrogen causes detrimental effects, such as reduced sperm production, cell division, and sculpting of the developing brain. These xenoestrogens are linked to the discovery that sperm counts worldwide plunged by 50 percent between 1938 and 1990. They are also linked to genital deformities; breast, prostate, and testicular cancer; and neurological disorders.[7]

Doctors see a consistent theme in women coming into their offices with complaints of the uncomfortable symptoms of PMS, perimenopause, and menopause. The effects come from too much estrogen, also known as estrogen dominance. Instead of estrogen playing its essential role within the well-balanced system of steroid hormones in our bodies, it has begun to overshadow the other pieces, creating a biochemical conflict.

The connection between what we put into our mouths and balancing our hormones is huge. Certain foods can decrease and increase estrogen in our bodies. Carbohydrates and refined sugars increase our insulin levels, which directly correlates to an increase in estrogen. We need to balance our insulin levels with some healthy fats and proteins.

Foods that impact your estrogen levels include flax, chia, alcohol, excess carbohydrates, and sugar. Also, what you put on your skin can cause bad estrogen. Increased bad estrogens can be caused by heating food in plastics, drinking from plastic water bottles, and using some scented candles and dryer sheets.

Follow these steps for managing estrogen levels:

- Cut estrogen-dominant foods, including flax, chia, soy, alcohol, and excess carbohydrates.

- Cut out sugar, which increases bad estrogen.

- Do not drink from plastic cups.

- Do not heat food in plastic containers or eat hot food from plastic plates.

- Stop putting chemicals on your skin, such as toxic makeup or lotions that cause estrogen dominance.

- Do not use scented candles or dryer sheets. Try reusable wool dryer balls instead!

- Consume adequate cholesterol and saturated fat. Cholesterol makes healthy hormones.

EFFECTS OF ESTROGEN DOMINANCE

- Excess estrogen usually means a progesterone deficiency. This deficiency leads to a decrease of new bone formation. Progesterone deficiency is the main cause of osteoporosis.

- When estrogen surpasses levels of progesterone, fat burning can be hindered (even with hard workouts) and weight can increase. Increased levels of estrogen cause headaches, irritability, chronic fatigue, and loss of interest in sex. These effects are also clinically recognized as premenstrual syndrome when our estrogen is naturally higher during menstrual cycles, which, for some women, are now happening for a whole month!

- Estrogen dominance promotes the development of breast cancer, but it also can cause fibrocystic breast disease. Estrogen levels can be balanced by adding a natural progesterone supplement.

- Estrogen dominance increases the risk of fibroids. One of the interesting facts about fibroids is that, regardless of the size, they commonly deteriorate once menopause arrives, and a woman's ovaries are no longer making estrogen.

- Endometrial cancer can develop.

- High blood pressure and hypertension are other scary side effects of estrogen dominance, which happens because there is water retention in the cells and an increase in intercellular sodium.

- Women with too much estrogen are at greater risk for heart disease and strokes.

- In men, estrogen dominance often results in prostate cancer and other issues.

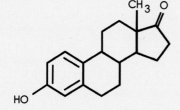

TESTOSTERONE

Most people think of testosterone as a male hormone, but women also have testosterone, which is needed for many functions. The amount of testosterone your body produces depends on your gender, age, diet, exercise habits, sleep patterns, menstrual cycle/menopause, stress levels, and any medications you're taking, as well as the time of day. In men, testosterone is produced in the testes; in women, the ovaries and adrenal glands produce testosterone. Unfortunately, levels decline with age.

Testosterone is essential for these six issues:

- Preserving muscle mass
- Facilitating sex drive
- Regulating moods
- Building energy
- Enhancing nutrition
- Forming masculine traits (in high levels)

Testosterone enhances muscle development, decreases fat stores, and increases bone mass. Testosterone and other hormones play an important role in determining your moods, depression, energy levels, ability to have orgasms, and ability to sleep.

Low testosterone levels have been directly linked to many undesirable health issues, including low sperm count, erectile dysfunction, low energy, mood changes, and weak bones. Low testosterone levels can increase body fat—particularly abdominal fat—and can cause deadly medical conditions, such as type 2 diabetes and heart disease. If you have low testosterone levels, your body easily burns muscle instead of fat and carbohydrates for fuel; often this situation is characterized by skinny legs and a bulging stomach.

So how do we hold onto our calorie-burning muscles? Muscles need protein. Hormones, like testosterone and human growth hormone, help proteins find their way to muscles and stay there. They also help preserve muscle once it has been made and help your body burn fat instead of muscle. If it wasn't for these hormones, protein from food could not create new muscles, and existing muscles would get quickly burned up for energy.

Low testosterone levels can be caused by many factors, including being overweight. A study in 2006 followed testosterone levels of 2,100 men age 45 and older. Researchers discovered that the obese men were 2.4 times more likely to have low testosterone compared to men who had a healthy weight.[8] Studies have also found that there is a direct connection to a decline of testosterone levels as body mass index (BMI) increases.

In general, weight loss can enhance testosterone. Researchers measured testosterone levels in two groups of middle-aged, obese

Statin Drugs Lead to Erectile Dysfunction

Statin drugs significantly lower hormones (especially testosterone) because statins lower cholesterol. Cholesterol is needed to make healthy hormones, which is why many men taking statins also take medication for erectile dysfunction.

men. One group followed a four-month weight-loss program, while the second group did nothing. The weight-loss group lost an average of 45 pounds and saw notable increases in testosterone levels compared to the second group, in which testosterone declined. More and more studies are linking body weight and testosterone levels. The human body has an intricate system of hormones that interact in a multitude of complex ways. The relationship between testosterone and weight is part of a large sequence of physiological processes that can be improved through diet and exercise.

We can't do anything about the natural progression of our biological clocks, but we can take control of our weight. Because testosterone production is known to decrease in direct proportion to the level of obesity, maintaining a healthy weight is critical.

Too little testosterone can lead to muscle loss, dry skin, poor skin elasticity, decreased libido, and bone density loss. Most people need to increase their levels of testosterone. Testosterone is lowered by alcohol, not getting enough protein, excess carbohydrates, and excess fat stores. Zinc is important for producing adequate testosterone. And what is high in zinc? That's right: beef and other animal proteins!

However, if you are a woman suffering from polycystic ovarian syndrome, keeping your testosterone levels low is important. Caffeine and sugar can increase these androgens (hormones that regulate fertility; elevated levels cause male characteristics such as dark facial hair) and should be avoided. The signs of too much testosterone include increased abdominal fat, acne, irregular periods, hair loss, irritability, and a decrease in breast size.

Follow these steps for managing testosterone levels:

- Cut out alcohol.
- Exercise! Lift heavy weights to stimulate testosterone.
- Lose weight. Weight loss increases testosterone.
- Eat adequate cholesterol and saturated fat to make healthy hormones.
- Eat beef; zinc produces testosterone.
- Do not consume flax, chia, or soy, all of which reduce testosterone.

DHEA

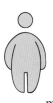

Scientists who study obesity recognize that losing excess weight is difficult. Indeed, the majority of dieters gain back unwanted weight, getting caught in endless cycles of yo-yo dieting. Researchers have concluded that the human body has a genetically determined set-point weight that is controlled by metabolic hormones.

One of these essential metabolic hormones is DHEA (dehydroepiandrosterone). DHEA is a steroid hormone that is produced by the adrenal glands. The body converts DHEA to male and female sex hormones, such as estrogen and testosterone. DHEA appears to have a stabilizing effect on all bodily systems. It also helps the body build lean muscle tissue.

As we age, our bodies produce less DHEA. Many scientists are now calling this hormone the "fountain of youth." DHEA levels peak at about age twenty; by age forty, we are producing half of the DHEA that we did at twenty. By age sixty-five, our bodies are producing about 15 percent of the DHEA we produced at twenty.[9] This decline has been linked to many common negative effects of aging as well as to many degenerative conditions, such as cancer, hardening of the arteries, a slowed immune system, memory loss, and a general lack of energy. These negative effects have led researchers to pay substantial attention to DHEA and its role in aging. In fact, DHEA supplements have been referred to as anti-aging hormones because people with lower levels of DHEA have been reported to suffer from adrenal deficiencies, kidney disease, type 2 diabetes, breast cancer, heart disease, and osteoporosis. Certain medications, such as corticosteroids, insulin, opiates, and danazol, also may deplete DHEA.

Our bodies have specific DHEA receptors, proving that DHEA affects us directly. DHEA is also in charge of stimulating hormones that control fat metabolism as well as stress. In general, DHEA is responsible for preserving vitality, leanness, and many other desirable traits associated with youth. Therefore, it seems likely that compensating for the decline in DHEA levels as we age would be of great benefit. By eating properly, we might find a way to reverse the aging process, essentially creating a "fountain of youth."

The U.S. Food and Drug Administration removed DHEA supplements from the market in 1985 because of false claims about health benefits. The U.S. Dietary Supplement Health and Education Act of 1994 returned these supplements to the market, and their popularity continues to grow. Despite this growth and attention, support for the health claims—particularly as tested on people—is lacking. Therefore, we want to bring your awareness to nutrition and how it can help increase and maintain DHEA levels.

You can naturally increase DHEA with exercise. Any type of exercise will help, but strength training really gets DHEA going.

Omega-3 fatty acids can play a big part in raising DHEA levels. Eat plenty of foods containing omega-3 fats, such as salmon and grass-fed meat.

Most people suffer from a magnesium deficiency. An adequate amount of magnesium increases the secretion of DHEA. Animal proteins (especially halibut) and leafy green vegetables are good sources of magnesium. A magnesium glycinate supplement just before bed is extremely beneficial, too. People used to get a lot of magnesium from their drinking water, but the proliferation of treated city water and bottled water has resulted in a loss of magnesium from our water supply, which means that many of us are deficient in magnesium and need to supplement.

Follow these steps for managing your DHEA levels:

- Consume fresh foods containing omega-3 fatty acids. Never take omega-3 supplements, which can easily become oxidized.
- Supplement with 400 to 800 milligrams of magnesium glycinate.
- Add exercise; strength training is best.
- Beware of medications that lower DHEA, such as corticosteroids, insulin, opiates, and danazol.
- Beware of DHEA supplements, which can affect any hormone, not just DHEA.

CORTISOL

Whenever we're anxious, angry, scared, or tense, our brains stimulate the production of cortisol and adrenaline, which are hormones designed to rouse the fight-or-flight response that was once essential to human survival. Adrenaline's role is to make you alert and focused. Cortisol increases your heart rate and tenses your muscles to get them ready to face the stressors ahead.

These physiological developments were important for our prehistoric ancestors, but they're not so helpful in a world where physical dangers are relatively few. Whenever we're stressed, our bodies release cortisol and adrenaline. Once the stress has passed, adrenaline levels fall, but cortisol remains high. Cortisol makes your body think that it needs to refuel as soon as possible because you've run a mile or done something physical in response to a "threat." Indulging in carbohydrate-loaded foods leads to weight gain and health issues for those who are chronically stressed. Eating carb-loaded foods can cause a blood sugar imbalance and can cause you to eat more than you need. It's a nasty cycle of stress, increased cortisol, junk food consumption, and weight gain!

The weight gain driven by this cycle is discouraging. Cortisol and adrenaline travel to fat cells, signaling them to open and release fat into the bloodstream, to the liver, and then to the muscles for use as energy. The scary problem is that fat cells deep inside the belly are particularly good at attracting cortisol. The cycle of hormonal responses caused by stress promotes the buildup of excess "stress fat" in the layer of fat below the abdominal muscle. Belly fat is the worst type of fat because it's "toxic weight"—the type of fat linked to heart disease, high blood pressure, stroke, cancer, and diabetes.

Unfortunately, in today's world, we all experience significant amounts of stress, and it doesn't appear to be going away anytime soon. Our daily lives naturally increase our cortisol levels. The things we do and put in our mouths every day can help keep this fat-storing hormone low. For some of us, our relationship with food just adds to already-elevated stress levels.

Although we can't totally eliminate external stress from our lives, there are some steps we can take to manage stress and keep our cortisol levels low:

- Limit consumption of carbs and sugar to stop that unpleasant belly fat from accumulating. Sugar is stressful for your body and can increase cortisol.

- Watch out for foods that can stimulate stress (carbohydrates and sugar), and concentrate on relaxing exercise, such as yoga, which is very effective at decreasing cortisol.

- Do your harder workouts in the morning when cortisol is naturally higher.

- Do not exercise or do intense workouts in the afternoon or evening when cortisol should be falling.

- Get eight to ten hours of restful sleep each night. When your adrenals are fatigued due to chronic stress, you need extra sleep, which is when the adrenals are restored. No adrenal supplement will help you if you aren't getting enough sleep and are working out like a cardio queen.

- Don't eat in stressful situations (working lunches and so forth), and limit relationships that cause stress.

- Simplify your life. Start saying no to others and *yes* to yourself! *Yes!*

- Try massage therapy and acupuncture to help relieve stress.

We hope the information in this chapter helps you better understand the roles that key hormones play in health and well-being. Getting our hormones balanced is one of the most rewarding things we can do for our health. A ketogenic diet goes a long way toward achieving that goal, but the steps outlined in this chapter can give your body the extra help it needs to return your hormones to a natural balance.

chapter 6

Modifications
for Disease

People are plagued by diseases today, and many suffer from multiple health conditions. A well-formulated ketogenic lifestyle will help you heal. If the damage that's already been done is severe, however, making some modifications to your diet and adding in some therapeutic supplements can be very helpful in speeding the healing process.

In this chapter, we examine a range of diseases and health conditions and give you both nutrition tweaks and suggestions for supplements that might help you heal faster.

CROHN'S DISEASE AND COLITIS

We see many clients with a variety of problems, including Crohn's disease and colitis. If Crohn's disease and ulcerative colitis are caught before considerable damage has been done, both conditions can be treated simply by restricting carbohydrates. As you know, carbs cause inflammation and prevent you from healing. When carbohydrates are limited, both Crohn's disease and ulcerative colitis respond rapidly. Carbohydrates, sugar, and vegetable oils are tremendously inflammatory and terrible for intestinal health.

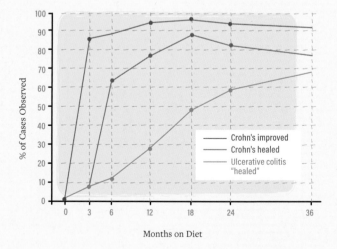

Red meat has long been wrongly blamed for these ailments. A study published in December 2009 shows that linoleic acid harms the gut, but news reports and health websites mislead the public by blaming red meat, which contains the least linoleic acid.[1] Polyunsaturated fats and oils, which are derived from seeds such as corn, soy, sunflower, and safflower, are the major dietary sources of linoleic acid. When linoleic acid is absorbed in the intestines, it is transformed into arachidonic acid, which is a component of the cell membranes in the bowel. Arachidonic acid can then be converted into various inflammatory compounds. High levels of these compounds have been found in the intestinal tissue of people suffering from intestinal disorders.

Fats from vegetable oils are found in prepackaged foods, salad dressings, roasted nuts, "baked" chips, popcorn, crackers, cereal—you name it! We have been wrongly pushed to replace healthy saturated fats like coconut oil with harmful fats such as canola oil.

Coconut oil is a medium-chain fatty acid (MCFA). MCFAs are broken down almost instantly by enzymes in the saliva and gastric juices so that pancreatic fat-digesting enzymes are not even important. The breakdown of MCFAs in saliva causes less strain on the pancreas and gastrointestinal system, which has significant benefits for people with intestinal issues. Because MCFA is easily absorbed in the digestive tract, it also helps other essential healing nutrients and supplements get absorbed. Ulcerative colitis often begins with a bacterial infection or virus that causes the body's immune system to malfunction and stays dynamic after the infection has cleared. Coconut has antimicrobial properties that help intestinal health by killing undesired microorganisms that cause chronic inflammation.

Our clients with the highest dietary intake of omega-3 fatty acid see the greatest reductions in difficulties from Crohn's disease and colitis. Omega-3 fatty acids are in oily fish such as salmon and sardines. However, skip the omega-3 supplements, which often go rancid and can do more harm than good.

 ## MODIFICATIONS

Cut out all dairy and nuts. However, unsweetened nut milks are okay.

Add cold therapy (see Chapter 12), which helps with gut disorders.

SUPPLEMENTS

Bifidobacteria: Make sure it is dairy-free and in the refrigerated section of your store. Keep it refrigerated, and take one capsule daily.

L-glutamine: Many hospitals now use L-glutamine to help healing (it heals intestinal lining and increases muscle strength). A healthy intestinal lining is crucial for healthy digestion, immune function, and liver health. Glutamine plays a major role in DNA synthesis and serves as a primary transporter of nitrogen into the muscle tissues. Take 3 grams thirty minutes before each meal.

Zinc: Zinc helps boost the immune system and is crucial for building proteins, utilizing enzymes, creating DNA, and helping cells communicate by acting as a neurotransmitter. We suggest 30 to 50 milligrams at breakfast, depending on how active you are and how much you sweat. The more you sweat, the more zinc you need. Note that zinc can cause nausea, so slowly increase your intake. Start with 10 milligrams a day for one week and then add 10 milligrams each week until you can take 50 milligrams per day without stomach upset.

HCl with pepsin: HCl features betaine HCl and the proteolytic enzyme pepsin, along with gentian root, which is an herbal bitter traditionally used to support digestion. Take one capsule with each meal.

SpectraZyme Pan 9X: SpectraZyme Pan 9X helps promote digestive function. The raw pancreatic enzymes contain proteases that break down protein, amylases that break down carbohydrates, and lipases that break down fat. Take one capsule with each meal.

Lipo-Gen: Lipo-Gen features a blend of fat metabolism nutrients including inositol, choline, and taurine. These nutrients are combined with methyl donors, folic acid, and vitamins B6 and B12, which help support liver function and bile flow. Take two capsules with each meal.

HIGH BLOOD PRESSURE

Most people who are insulin resistant also have high blood pressure. Insulin resistance is directly caused by a high-sugar, high-grain (even complex carbs) diet. High blood pressure and uncontrolled blood sugar go hand in hand. Typically, as insulin increases, so does blood pressure. Insulin stores magnesium, but if your insulin receptors are resistant and your cells grow resistant to insulin, you can't store magnesium, so magnesium passes out of your body through urination. Magnesium in your cells relaxes your muscles. If your magnesium level is too low, your blood vessels constrict rather than relax, which raises your blood pressure and decreases your energy level. Most Americans are deficient in magnesium.

Insulin also affects your blood pressure by causing your body to retain sodium. Sodium retention causes fluid retention. Fluid retention, in turn, causes high blood pressure and can lead to congestive heart failure.

To enhance your heart health, first remove all grains and sugars, especially fructose, from your diet until your blood pressure and weight are under control (and insulin signaling is thus restored). Eating sugar and grains—including any bread, pasta, corn, potatoes, or rice—will cause your insulin levels and your blood pressure to rise.

Fructose is a sugar that can be metabolized only by the liver; the liver breaks down the fructose into a variety of waste products—including uric acid—that are unhealthy for your body. Uric acid drives up your blood pressure by inhibiting the nitric oxide in your blood vessels. Nitric oxide helps your vessels maintain their elasticity, so nitric oxide suppression leads to increases in blood pressure.

MODIFICATIONS

Eat keto and avoid all foods that boost insulin levels. Even whole grains rapidly break down to sugars. Complex carbs are just glucose molecules joined together in long chains.

Balance your omega-6 to omega-3 fat ratio. Most people eating a standard American diet have a ratio omega-6 to omega-3 fats of 25:1, which is super-unbalanced. The ideal ratio is 1:1. To achieve this ratio, reduce the amount of vegetable oil in your diet and consume foods that contain high-quality, animal-based sources of omega-3s.

SUPPLEMENTS

Vitamin D: Healthy vitamin D levels can have a strong effect on normalizing blood pressure. Low levels are associated with an increased risk of heart disease. Vitamin D has a positive effect on diabetes. You can get a blood test to check your vitamin D levels. If your level is lower than 45, get some sun exposure and consider taking a supplement; we recommend 1,000 IU per 25 pounds of body weight to maintain vitamin D levels. However, try to keep your vitamin D level lower than 70. Make sure you take vitamin D while eating a food that contains fat because vitamin D is fat soluble, and every cell in your body has a vitamin D receptor.

Magnesium glycinate: Many people are deficient in magnesium because our food and water supplies don't contain the levels of magnesium they once did, so a supplement is necessary for most people. If you supplement magnesium, you need to take a very absorbable form of magnesium. We recommend 400 milligrams of magnesium glycinate when you wake because blood pressure is highest in the morning. (Do not use magnesium oxide or citrate because it will just cause loose stools.) Take another 400 milligrams just before bed to help your blood vessels relax.

L-carnitine: L-carnitine helps increase energy, weight loss, and focus, and it decreases triglycerides. It is an amino acid that shuttles fatty acids into the mitochondria—the "fat-burning powerhouses" in your body. Also, L-carnitine helps restrict the buildup of fat around the liver and heart. Take 3 grams in the morning on an empty stomach; taking L-carnitine later in the day can affect your sleep.

CoQ10: This is a coenzyme that increases mitochondria building. It is in the mitochondria where fat is oxidized, which keeps cells and liver more sensitized to insulin. Take 400 milligrams of CoQ10 with the first meal of the day.

KEEP AN EYE ON YOUR BLOOD PRESSURE

Make sure to watch your blood pressure. As you eat keto and add in supplements, your blood pressure will go down, and you might be able to stop taking blood pressure medications. Always work with your healthcare professional to monitor your levels and adjust medications as needed.

THYROID

We all want to blame our thyroid when it comes to weight gain. However, studies show that a sluggish thyroid isn't going to make us gain 100 pounds; a malfunctioning thyroid is responsible for only 5 to 12 pounds of weight gain. In addition to affecting weight gain, the thyroid contributes to how well we sleep, produces stomach acid, can cause high cholesterol, and helps with absorption of nutrients. Your weight might not be the only issue affected by your thyroid; there are some other serious issues that can be caused by thyroid problems.

It is extremely important to know what is causing the thyroid issue before you begin taking any medication prescribed by a doctor. If you have an autoimmune disorder, adjusting your diet is an important factor in addressing the root cause of the disease. If you do decide to take medication, then you should also eat correctly while taking the medication. Doing so allows your body to control the autoimmune response, which will affect the dosage you need of the medication. Once you address and eliminate what is causing the autoimmune response, you can likely lower the dose.

Bone loss and other issues can happen if you take too much thyroid hormone and your TSH falls below 1.5. Inflammation is a primary cause of bone loss, which is why you need to address your diet first.

Cellular hypothyroidism, which is when thyroid hormone levels decrease, can be brought on by chronic physical or emotional stress. Chronic disease, adrenal fatigue, and low ferritin levels can also cause cellular hypothyroidism.

In 90 percent of cases, hypothyroidism (Hashimoto's thyroiditis) is an autoimmune disease. Autoimmune diseases like Hashimoto's disease and Graves' disease are likely caused by a gluten and/or dairy intolerance. Here's what happens: A healthy thyroid stimulates the production of hydrochloric acid (stomach acid). When the thyroid is underperforming, stomach acid is reduced, which causes food to sit in the stomach too long, resulting in perforations (holes) in the gut lining. Holes in the intestinal lining leads to leaky gut, which causes food to enter the bloodstream. Leaky gut allows food to leak into the bloodstream. The body doesn't recognize these foreign substances, causing an autoimmune response. In other words, your blood doesn't know

> "
>
> *I can't thank you enough for all your help, Maria! After 27 years of uncontrolled Hashimoto's disease, my thyroid is now normal without Synthroid. My doctor still runs tests every six months because she's never seen a thyroid recover like mine has after quitting grains and sugar.*
>
> —Sharon

Allergy Tests Are Often Inaccurate

Many people make the mistake of running to the doctor for an allergy blood test to determine whether a food allergy is the cause of their problems. Unfortunately, we believe blood tests are very inaccurate. This claim might sound crazy, but we believe it to be true. Some of our clients with autoimmune diseases can no longer produce antibodies because their immune systems are worn out. We believe everyone should kick gluten regardless of antibody test results.

what the substances are, and it puts your immune system into overdrive to kill the foreign substances. The antibodies produced to attack gliadin and other foreign substances in the blood also attack the thyroid. If you continue to eat gluten, your immune system continues to attack your thyroid. We recommend that our clients get thyroid antibody tests, which help determine whether there is a food allergy.

Some of our clients mistakenly think they can eat small amounts of bread or gluten on the weekends or at social gatherings, but they can't. The immune response to gluten can last up to six months every time you consume it. Gluten isn't an 80/20 issue in which you can follow the rules only 80 percent of the time. You must remove 100 percent of food allergens to stop the immune response from occurring.

MODIFICATIONS

Cut out all gluten, dairy, and soy.

SUPPLEMENTS

HCl with pepsin: A healthy thyroid produces stomach acid. If you are deficient in hydrochloric acid, you can't absorb the nutrients for bone health and thyroid function. A helpful supplement is 500 to 700 milligrams of HCl with pepsin before meals.

Zinc: You lose a lot of zinc through sweat. A deficiency in zinc can lead to low thyroid, acne, low testosterone, hair loss, eye and skin lesions, impaired appetite, and low immune function. A zinc deficiency causes cravings for salt or for a bite of sweetness after a meal. We suggest 30 to 50 milligrams at breakfast. Zinc can cause nausea, so increase your intake gradually. Start with 10 milligrams

Autoimmune-Triggering Foods and Thyroidectomies

Have you had a thyroidectomy? If so, you still need to eliminate autoimmune-triggering foods because a thyroidectomy is like removing gum from the bottom of your shoe; even after you get rid of most of the gum, a little bit remains. Because the thyroid is located in a vulnerable area, there will still be some thyroid present after the thyroidectomy. In the case of cancerous or noncancerous nodules, there will still be antibody production against the small amount of thyroid that's left if you continue to eat gluten and dairy. You need to address the foods causing autoimmune responses by cutting out all dairy and gluten.

a day for one week and then add 10 milligrams each week until you can take 50 milligrams a day without stomach upset.

L-tyrosine: L-tyrosine is essential for supporting the processes affected by thyroid hormone and epinephrine (adrenaline); it also supports healthy glandular function and adrenal/stress response. Tyrosine is an amino acid naturally found in animal products such as red meat. Tyrosine can also be produced by phenylalanine, another amino acid, but it needs iron for conversion. Often, women lack iron because food allergies inhibit their ability to absorb it. Women also might lack iron because they don't eat red meat, endure heavy periods, or have uterine fibroids. These issues can cause them to be unable to make tyrosine, and they often end up with low thyroid function. Some of our clients who are suffering from stress end up with low thyroid because they require more tyrosine to deal with stressors. Take 1,000 milligrams first thing in the morning and another 1,000 milligrams mid-morning.

Iodine: If you are using a quality sea salt, you likely are not getting any iodine. (Table salt is fortified with iodine.) All hormones need iodine to function. More than 80 percent of the U.S. population is deficient in iodine, which causes poor circulation. Symptoms of

WHITE SPOTS ON NAILS = LOW ZINC

Do you have white spots on your nails? We had a client who was taking 50 milligrams of zinc a day for more than two years and still showed signs of low zinc, which include white spots on the nails. She had been on thyroid medication for years, but her doctor never addressed how the thyroid can affect digestion and absorption. The thyroid is a zinc "hog" and needs more than what you can get from a typical diet (unless you love oysters and beef, which are high in zinc).

iodine deficiency are feeling cold; feeling sluggish and tired; having difficulty losing weight; and suffering from dry skin, hair loss, constipation, and miscarriages. Children with iodine deficiency can have impaired brain development. Note that you lose 52 milligrams of iodine from one hour of sweating. To supplement iodine, take 325 milligrams in the form of kelp.

Selenium: Selenium is essential for the conversion of T4 to T3, which is the active form of thyroid hormone. During pregnancy, the immune system goes into overdrive to protect the fetus. Once the baby is born, the mother develops antibodies against the thyroid. Taking selenium while pregnant is very safe and helps lower the autoimmune response that often happens after giving birth. Take 200 micrograms once a day.

Vitamin D: Take 1,000 IU per 25 pounds of body weight. Try to keep your levels between 45 and 70.

Gamma-linoleic acid (GLA): Gamma-linoleic acid and linoleic acid are essential for skin health, skin elasticity, and cellular structure. These fatty acids regulate hormones, including thyroid and sex hormones. These hormones improve nerve function, which lowers pain from fibromyalgia, PMS, and migraine headaches. For women, we recommend getting GLA via emu oil. Take 1,500 milligrams of emu oil or 1,300 milligrams of evening primrose oil three times a day with food. Men should take borage oil; supplement with 600 milligrams of borage oil three times a day, preferably with food.

EstroFactors: This supplement detoxes bad estrogen from the liver. Anything that impairs liver function or ties up the detoxifying function results in excess estrogen levels, or estrogen dominance. Take three capsules a day for one month, and then switch to one capsule per day ongoing with food. (EstroFactors contains some vitamin A, which is fat soluble and is better metabolized with food.)

Estrogen Dominance Leads to Cancer

Did you know that thyroid cancer is an estrogen-dominant cancer? Yep! Breast, uterine, ovarian, and prostate cancers also are estrogen-dominant. Even men can have estrogen dominance.

GETTING OFF THYROID MEDICATION

Work with a healthcare professional to watch your thyroid numbers closely if you are on medication for a slow thyroid and you start eating keto, eliminating common food allergens, and adding thyroid-supporting supplements. Many of our clients have been able to stop taking their thyroid medication within weeks.

GOUT

Outbreaks of gout have doubled over the last twenty-five years. This painful ailment occurs when uric acid builds up and forms into sharp, needle-like urate crystals. These crystals lodge in soft tissues and the extremity joints, such as the big toes. Gout causes inflammation, swelling, and terrible pain.

Gout is most commonly treated with a diet that is low in protein and high in fructose. In reality, though, this approach causes even more problems.

Uric acid is a breakdown of protein compounds known as purines, which are the building blocks of amino acids. High concentrations of purines are found in meat, so doctors assumed that the primary cause of elevated uric acid levels in the blood is excessive meat consumption.

The actual cause is quite shocking. Just as a low-sodium diet has been proven not to help with lowering blood pressure, and a cholesterol-free diet doesn't help with decreasing heart disease, a low-purine diet does not affect uric acid levels! For example, we had a client who was doing great on the ketogenic diet. Then she traveled to Peru, where she gorged on high-sugar fruits, such as bananas, mangoes, and pineapple. She called to say that she was suffering from extreme pain in her big toe. Yep, it was gout. The enormous amount of fructose was causing elevated uric acid levels. Her doctor advised her to follow a vegetarian diet, which only worsened her problems because she was eating a lot of fruit filled with fructose. A vegetarian diet drops serum uric acid levels

Lowering Liver Enzymes with Castor Oil and Zendocrine

T4 is converted to the activated T3 in the liver, not in the thyroid. Get your liver enzymes checked (via a blood test) if you have a thyroid disorder causing a low T3 level but have a normal T4 level. If your liver enzymes are elevated, use castor oil packs at least two or three times a week. Add a drop of dōTERRA Zendocrine oil (a combination of tangerine peel, rosemary leaf, geranium plant, juniper berry, and cilantro herb essential oils) to some castor oil and rub the combination on your liver area (lower-right abdomen). Cover the area with some wool flannel, a towel, and a hot water bottle for at least forty-five minutes once a day. Another option is milk thistle, which can also cleanse the liver.

by about 10 percent compared to a typical American diet, but that doesn't decrease uric acid buildup very much, and the extreme pain doesn't go away.

Another shocking piece of the puzzle is that eating additional protein increases the excretion of uric acid from the kidneys, which decreases the level of uric acid in the blood. Therefore, high-protein diets are helpful, even if the purines aren't.

So if eating protein doesn't actually cause gout, what does? Insulin resistance! Insulin resistance increases uric acid levels because uric acid elimination by the kidneys is decreased. Insulin resistance also raises blood pressure by decreasing sodium excretion. Cutting carbs from your diet will help heal your gout. A ketogenic diet, which reduces carb consumption and helps lower insulin levels, helps heal gout.

One specific carbohydrate source you should avoid at all costs is fructose. Fructose causes many problems, but we now know that it also is a primary contributor to gout because it increases serum levels of uric acid. The connection between fructose and gout was first written about in the journal *The Lancet* in the late 1960s. The study proved fructose accelerated the breakdown of ATP (adenosine triphosphate)—the primary source of energy—and it is loaded with purines.[2] Adenosine is a form of adenine, and adenine is a purine, which increases production of uric acid. Alcohol also raises uric acid levels through the same reaction.

Fructose also stimulates the production of purines. The metabolism of fructose leads the body to produce lactic acid, which inhibits the excretion of uric acid by the kidneys, which in turn raises uric acid levels.

Keep in mind that natural foods—even fruits—contain fructose. Excess fructose comes from table sugar, honey, high-fructose corn syrup, and agave. Table sugar is about 50 percent fructose, honey is about 55 percent fructose, high-fructose corn syrup can be up to 65 percent fructose, and agave is about 90 percent fructose! In the presence of extreme health conditions, you should avoid these natural sources of fructose.

MODIFICATIONS

Cut out all fructose as well as alcohol.

GOUT CAN BE CAUSED BY A GENETIC DEFECT

There is a genetic defect that can make gout run in families. This defect causes a difficulty in metabolizing fructose and a predisposition to gout if too much fructose is consumed.

ACID REFLUX AND INDIGESTION

We can't help but notice that everywhere we turn we see acid-blocking medications being sold. Prescription drugs for acid reflux have serious consequences, and the directions clearly state that they are not to be used for longer than two weeks. However, they are sold in America like the candy they're shelved next to. When we work with clients in other countries, acid blockers are not easy to come by, and patients are allowed to take them only for two weeks at a time. However, today, we are seeing clients put on these meds long-term—and not just adults, but babies, too! In most cases, acid reflux is caused by not having enough stomach acid, not by having too much.

We'll never forget our client Sara. She was the mother of a six-month-old who was on acid blockers. Her baby girl didn't get better after starting one acid blocker, so you know what the doctor did? Gave her another acid blocker to take in addition to the first! This poor baby was on two acid blockers with no action plan for how to heal her gut. The doctor said Sara's daughter would most likely need to take acid blockers for her whole life! After we changed the baby's diet, she was off both acid blockers within days. We cut out rice cereals, fruit, and dairy and replaced those items with bone broth, mashed avocados, mashed egg yolks, bone marrow, and other baby-friendly keto foods.

In case you're wondering what's wrong with taking acid blockers for your whole life, let us tell you about our client Bill. At age eighteen, Bill started taking acid blockers. When he came

ACID REFLUX IS NOT NORMAL

When I was sixteen, I went to see my family physician because I couldn't eat anything without suffering from acid reflux. She chuckled and stated, "I get it when I drink water!" My doctor acted as if acid reflux was a normal reaction after eating. At the time, I had a lot of respect for doctors and believed that they were always right, so I thought my acid reflux wasn't a big deal. She suffered from it, too, so it must be okay to have acid reflux. Now I sit back and remember that moment with frustration. My doctor never asked what I ate when I got acid reflux, but that's because she didn't—and still doesn't—connect diet with how our bodies respond to the foods we eat. I now know that starting the day with whole-grain cereal and milk was a recipe for disaster.

to us, he was thirty-five and suffered every time he ate. Taking acid blockers for long periods causes more issues than you could ever imagine. In Bill's case, his intestines resembled Swiss cheese because of all the holes that had formed in lining. Whenever Bill ate, undesired food particles leached into his bloodstream, where they shouldn't be; this is known as leaky gut. As a result, his autoimmune system went into overdrive and caused an autoimmune response. Acid blockers can agitate a range of autoimmune disorders, including rheumatoid arthritis, multiple sclerosis, Hashimoto's thyroiditis, Graves' disease, and many more.

Antacids cause ulcers, chronic inflammation, leaky gut, food allergies, anemia, inflammatory bowel disease, digestive issues, and restless leg syndrome. The stomach is a very acidic environment with a pH of 2 or less. Stomach acid is essential for absorbing vitamin B12 and minerals that allow you to release hormones from the pancreas; without these hormones, you can develop diabetes. Stomach acid also helps break down protein. When you don't have stomach acid to break down food, undigested protein sits like a rock in your intestines. This undigested protein slowly eats holes in your intestines, and the inflammation begins a detrimental snowball effect. When you have holes in your intestines, food starts to leak into your bloodstream (leading to leaky gut). Leaky gut causes the immune system to go into overdrive to kill the unknown substances in the blood, and you enter the world of food allergies! When this happens, other health issues follow, such as chronic and seasonal allergies, constipation and/or diarrhea, and inflammatory bowel diseases.

There are many natural ways to clear acid reflux without side effects.

HEALING ACID REFLUX

Hydrochloric acid (HCl) is a digestive juice produced in the stomach that breaks down nutrients and stimulates numerous enzymes and hormones. A decrease of HCl is related to acid reflux and reduced function of the digestive system. If you have been taking acid blockers, you're not producing HCl in suitable amounts needed to break down foods. Production of HCl declines with age, and it also can lead to an inability to taste food. Coffee, alcohol, antacids, and cigarettes all contribute to the excessive

GUT DAMAGE

My dad has been on acid blockers for years. Sadly, when he travels to other countries, he often gets sick from food poisoning or parasites. If your gut is healthy, your body can fight off bad bacteria. However, if your gut is damaged and you have low levels of good gut bacteria, you are more susceptible to illnesses and parasites.

production of hydrochloric acid, which can eventually "wear out" the stomach's ability to produce it. Also, thyroid disorders and emotional distress can cause low HCl. That means you should reduce or eliminate coffee, alcohol, antacid use, smoking, and stress. Taking care of your gut by eliminating harmful substances is the first step to recovery; eventually, your stomach's ability to function optimally will be restored.

Follow these guidelines for resolving acid reflux:

- Chew your food well—thirty-two times before swallowing.
- Eat only when you are hungry, and never when you are upset, as it can impair digestion.
- Do not drink while eating. Liquids dilute your digestive enzymes.
- Skip coffee, carbonated beverages, alcohol, and aspirin, which contribute to damage of the intestinal wall.
- Cut out dairy and gluten, which are common allergens. Decrease your intake of foods containing chemicals, vegetable oils, sugar, and starch. If you are suffering from a food allergy or sensitivity, eliminate gluten and dairy or the food that causes the acid reflux.
- Eat foods that heal the intestines, such as coconut oil, bone broth, and gelatin.
- Get your thyroid checked. A healthy thyroid produces HCl. If your thyroid is slow, relieving acid reflux could be as simple as adding HCl.
- Use high-quality sea salt, which is something many of our clients neglect to do. We recommend eliminating processed table salt in favor of an unprocessed salt, such as Celtic or Himalayan sea salt. These unprocessed salts provide you with more than eighty trace minerals that you need to perform optimally; and they help your body support you biochemically to naturally produce HCl.

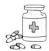 ## SUPPLEMENTS

Bifidobacteria: Supplement with a high-quality probiotic that includes *Bifidobacteria* as well as acidophilus. *Bifidobacteria* helps balance your bowel flora, which naturally can help eliminate

Helicobacter (also known as *H. pylori*, an overgrowth of bad gut bacteria). A healthy gut contains good bacteria in the digestive tract that helps digest food and combat harmful invaders. These healthy bacteria release compounds that we can then absorb and make use of, such as vitamins D and K2. Acid reflux can often be caused by *H. pylori*, a pathogenic organism; it's the only bacterial organism in the stomach that is never killed by hydrochloric acid. Probiotics can attack *H. pylori* and other harmful organisms.

L-glutamine: Glutamine plays a major role in DNA synthesis and serves as a primary transporter of nitrogen into the muscle tissues. It also decreases sugar, carbs, and alcohol cravings. Time and time again, studies have shown that a therapeutic dose of supplemental glutamine shields against gastric lesions and helps heal aching ulcers. In fact, cabbage juice, which is very high in glutamine, is a folk remedy for ulcers. Take 3 grams of L-glutamine about fifteen minutes before each meal.

Zinlori: Zinlori is a patented zinc-carnosine complex that helps the ecology of the gut by increasing its natural defenses and boosting the cellular integrity of the intestinal lining. Take one capsule on an empty stomach twice a day.

Hydrochloric acid: HCl helps your body digest your food and absorb nutrients; it also kills Helicobacter and decreases uncomfortable symptoms that result from too much of the bacteria. Take one to three capsules every time you eat. Betaine HCl supplements are available in health food stores without a prescription. You'll want to take as many as you need to get the slightest burning sensation and then decrease by one capsule.

Aloe vera: Aloe vera naturally repairs the damage to the esophagus safely. Aloe vera's major ingredient buffers pH+ and speeds the healing process. The aloe will put a protective coating on the esophagus and helps control reflux. Take one to three capsules (10,000 milligrams each) three times a day.

Vitamin D: Your vitamin D levels are important because there is often an infectious component to gastrointestinal issues. Optimizing your vitamin D levels also stimulates your production of 200 antimicrobial peptides that will protect you and help your body eradicate infections. Increase your sun exposure and consider

Gradually Reduce Acid Blockers

If you have been on acid blockers for longer than two weeks, you can't stop cold turkey. Getting off acid blockers is a transition. The first steps are to add the following supplements while cutting out dairy, gluten, and carbs. After you've started the supplements and modified your diet, then (and only then) cut your medication by one-quarter; continue that dose for a week. Then cut your dose by another quarter and take that for a week. At the beginning of the third week, cut your medication by another quarter for one week.

taking a vitamin D supplement. If you take vitamin D, always take 100 to 200 micrograms of vitamin K2 as well. If your vitamin D levels are below 45, take 1,000 IU per 25 pounds of body weight with a meal (vitamin D is fat-soluble).

GALLBLADDER REMOVAL

A question we get almost daily is, "Can I eat keto if I no longer have a gallbladder?"

Recently, we were interviewed by a popular newspaper, and the interviewer asked if a person whose gallbladder had been removed could eat keto. Yes, the keto diet is good for someone without a gallbladder. The common bile duct, which remains after the gallbladder is removed, takes over much of the gallbladder's function when the gallbladder is taken out, which is why people who've had theirs removed can still digest fat. Coconut oil and MCT oil are very good for people who've had their gallbladders removed because they don't require bile acids for absorption.

MODIFICATIONS

Cut out all dairy. Everyone should cut out vegetable oils, but doing so is especially crucial if you do not have a gallbladder.

SUPPLEMENTS

Dandelion and ox bile: Add dandelion and ox bile to increase bile production.

Lipo-Gen: Lipo-Gen is a brand of supplement that features fat metabolism–enhancing nutrients, including taurine, inositol, and choline. These nutrients are combined with methyl donors, folic acid, and vitamins B6 and B12, which help support bile flow and healthy liver function. Take two capsules of Lipo-Gen with meals.

SpectraZyme Pan 9X: This product is a complex enzyme that boosts digestive function. The raw pancreatic enzyme contains proteases to break down protein, amylases to break down carbohydrates, and lipases to break down fat. SpectraZyme contains whole, raw peptidases, nucleases, and elastases. Take one capsule of SpectraZyme Pan 9X with a meal.

GASTRIC BYPASS

We have had many clients who have gone through gastric bypass surgery, which comes with many side effects, such as poor mineral absorption and low iron. Often clients tell us they wish they would have known about the ketogenic diet before they'd had such a drastic surgery.

MODIFICATIONS

Skip the veggies, which just take up space needed for nutrient-dense protein. Your protein intake needs to increase after gastric bypass because your body absorbs less protein. Preserving muscle mass is essential when losing weight.

Consider doing a protein-sparing modified fast (see page 88) twice per week.

Skip the calcium supplements that bariatric doctors always recommend. Calcium supplements are poorly absorbed and can cause calcification of the arteries.

SUPPLEMENTS

Iron: You might need liquid iron because your iron absorption is poor. However, make sure you are low in iron before you begin taking supplements. Never take iron supplements unless you know you are low. Work with a healthcare professional to determine what dose to take and when to take it based on your current iron levels.

HCl: Take one or two HCl capsules (500 to 600 milligrams each) with each meal to increase the absorption of nutrients and reduce indigestion.

ACNE, ECZEMA, AND OTHER SKIN ISSUES

Using antibiotics for acne is unnecessary because eliminating sugar and carbs creates an internal environment that does not allow for bacterial overgrowth. Taking antibiotics is detrimental to your gut flora because it kills all your good gut bacteria, which can lead to a compromised gut, autoimmune diseases, and food allergies.

Other skin issues, like eczema, can be caused by excess sugars as well, but they also can be caused by a sensitivity to gluten or dairy. Eliminating grains and dairy along with sugar can be an important step in reversing a wide range of skin issues.

MODIFICATIONS

Avoid simple carbohydrates. By now, you know that simple carbohydrates—bread, rice, soda, candy, cookies, and all sugars— are just empty calories. The first step to clearing up your skin is to eliminate simple carbs. Ridding your refrigerators and pantries of high-fructose corn syrup is a step we all should take. We should also teach our kids how to read labels so that they never consume high-fructose corn syrup. (It's even in some pickles!) Fructose is metabolized by the liver and contributes to fatty liver disease. Fresh fruit also contains a large amount of fructose, so you should consume it in very limited amounts and never in the form of juice.

Steer clear of mold. You should avoid *Candida*, meaning no mushrooms, peanut butter, or mold products (including cheese and marijuana). Get your house checked for black mold as well.

Avoid complex carbohydrates. Complex carbs are just glucose molecules linked together in long chains; our bodies break them down into glucose (sugar) in our blood. Complex carbohydrates are in foods such as beans, nuts, whole grains, and starchy vegetables. These foods sound healthy, right? However, limiting these foods will decrease the inflammation of the skin caused by the rise in insulin. High insulin levels increase male androgen hormones (yes, even in women), which makes your pores secrete excess sebum, a greasy material that traps acne-promoting bacteria. This rise in androgens also causes polycystic ovary syndrome (PCOS) and fertility issues, so a keto diet would greatly help women suffering from PCOS. Insulin also causes skin cells to multiply, a progression connected to acne.

Avoid gluten. Gluten is a leading cause of rosacea and causes acne; gluten can push toxins through the skin, which causes skin ailments. However, you must be careful when choosing gluten-free products, such as gluten-free bread and anything that contains rice flour, tapioca starch, or other high-carb ingredients, which won't help lower inflammation of the skin. You might think it's

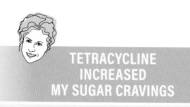

TETRACYCLINE INCREASED MY SUGAR CRAVINGS

I remember being put on tetracycline for acne when I was fourteen years old. Sure, the medication cleared up my acne, but it also put my sugar cravings into overdrive.

impossible to be keto and eat gluten-free and low-carb, but we do it, and we still enjoy foods like pizza, donuts, and risotto; we just enjoy keto-modified versions!

Detox bad estrogens. (This includes men and boys!) Our bodies produce three types of estrogen:

- The ovaries produce healthy estrogen—estradiol.
- Fat cells store and form unhealthy estrogen—estrone.
- Women's bodies produce estriol when pregnant.

The scary truth is that estrogen comes from our food. Our bodies make more estrogen when we eat too many processed carbohydrates, drink alcohol, or consume flax and chia. The pancreas secrete insulin, the master hormone, in response to sugar and processed carbs. Insulin stores fat and causes our bodies to make more estrogen. Don't microwave food in plastic or drink from plastic bottles. Purchase hormone-free meat and eggs. Topical products, scented candles, and dryer sheets can also increase bad estrogen.

Eliminate dairy. Dairy can cause red bumps, acne, and other inflammatory skin disorders.

SUPPLEMENTS

Bifidobacteria: A healthy gut contains good bacteria in the digestive tract, which helps digest food and combat harmful invaders. These healthy bacteria release compounds—such as vitamins D and K2—that we can then absorb and make use of. Taking antibiotics for the treatment of acne also kills good gut bacteria, which can cause *Candida* overgrowth and increase skin outbreaks. Supplement with a high-quality probiotic that includes *Bifidobacteria,* and take it in the morning before you eat. For most people, one capsule a day is an appropriate amount. If you are taking antibiotics or have a recovering immune system, take two or three capsules a day until your gut health is restored, then drop to one capsule per day. Loose stools are a sign you should back down to one capsule a day.

Zinc: If you are an athlete or you sweat a lot, you are likely low in zinc. This often causes "backne" (acne on the upper back). Adding zinc boosts your immune system to combat the bacteria that causes the acne. Zinc can cause nausea, so start with 10 milligrams a day for one week. Increase by 10 milligrams each week until you can take 50 milligrams in a single dose without feeling nauseated.

Iodine: We recommend using a high-quality sea salt instead of traditional table salt. However, sea salt isn't fortified with iodine (as table salt is), and more than 80 percent of Americans are deficient. All our hormones need iodine to function. Iodine deficiency causes us to feel sluggish and tired, makes losing weight difficult, and causes dry skin, acne, hair loss, constipation, cold sensitivity, and poor brain development in children. We suggest taking 325 milligrams in the form of a kelp supplement once a day with food.

Gamma-linoleic acid (GLA): The gamma-linoleic acid and linoleic acid are essential for skin health, elasticity of the skin, and cellular structure. These fatty acids regulate hormones, including the thyroid and sex hormones. They improve nerve function and reduce pain from fibromyalgia, PMS, and migraine headaches. Women should take 1,500 milligrams of emu oil or 1,300 milligrams of evening primrose oil three times daily, with food. Men should take borage oil; supplement with 600 milligrams of borage oil three times a day, preferably with food.

EstroFactors: This supplement detoxes bad estrogen from the liver that can cause acne. Anything that impairs liver function or ties up the detoxifying function will result in excess estrogen levels. Take three capsules a day for a month, and then take one capsule per day with food. (The capsules contain some vitamin A, which is fat soluble and will digest better with food.)

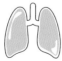

D-HIST: D-HIST is a natural d-histamine; you can find it at health food stores or online. D-HIST helps with sinus issues and skin rashes. Also, high histamine levels block serotonin from being absorbed, which often causes depression. If you have high histamine levels, add one to three capsules daily with food.

ASTHMA

Inflammation of the lungs is caused by sugar, starch, complex carbohydrates, food allergies, and trans fats. Inflammation of the lungs causes asthma.

Starchy foods (even complex carbohydrates) are just glucose molecules hooked together in long chains, and they increase blood

sugar levels. (Yeast loves sugar!) Sugar and starchy foods cause
the blood sugar to upsurge quickly and then plummet to a lower-
than-normal level. The upswing intensifies the problem; the drop
in blood sugar causes the production of serotonin to decrease and
causes depression. The decrease in serotonin causes the production
of histamine, which leads to the enlargement of blood vessels.
Overexpansion of blood vessels causes liquid in the vessels to seep
out. When liquid seeps out into the sinus area, it results in a nasal
drip. Asthma can be caused when the sinus drips into the bronchii.
When it drips into the brain, it causes headaches and migraines.

MODIFICATIONS

Cut out foods high in histamines. We suggest that you steer clear of
fruit; even low-sugar strawberries have a high histamine response.

SUPPLEMENTS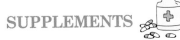

Magnesium glycinate: Many mineral deficiencies can cause
asthma. The most common deficiency we see is magnesium, which
is most likely the most important mineral for decreasing asthma
because of its powerful effect on relaxing the bronchial muscle.
This subsequently causes a reduction of bronchospasm and
increases the airway's diameter. Magnesium reduces the histamine
response, which also calms inflammation. Our clients who suffer
from asthma often have high histamine release from white blood
cells, which causes inflammation and bronchoconstriction. Quality
magnesium supplements dull this response. Magnesium increases
the production of AMP and ATP, two significant mediators that
generate relaxation of bronchospasm. If you supplement with
magnesium, you need to take a very absorbable form. Take 400
milligrams before bed and another 400 milligrams in the morning.

D-HIST: D-HIST is a natural d-histamine. You can find D-HIST at
health food stores or online. It will not only help with sinus issues
but also clear up skin rashes. High histamines block serotonin
from being absorbed and often cause depression. If you have high
histamine levels, take one capsule of D-HIST twice a day with food.

DEPRESSION, ANXIETY, AND OTHER MOOD ISSUES

Can depression be caused by diet? Yes. Serotonin is used mainly in your gut: 80 to 90 percent is found there; the rest is in your brain. This is why the food we eat is so important. Serotonin controls appetite, hormones, sleep, mood, and anger. Serotonin deficiency is a primary cause of depression. Serotonin is one of the more well-studied neurotransmitters because it affects your personality in such a profound way. It is the brain's natural antidepressant.

Two of the most common serious ailments we see in our office are depression and anxiety. Low serotonin levels cause your body to crave carbohydrates and sweets. Carbohydrates increase insulin in your bloodstream. When you eat carbs or sweets, insulin then rewards you with an extreme feeling of gratification. Your brain is screaming for this gratification, but not for long. Soon after the carbohydrate binge, your serotonin diminishes, and the cycle continues. Eating sweet and carbohydrate-laden foods in an attempt to relieve the cravings leads to weight gain and a fatty

WE ARE WHAT WE EAT

Before I started my job as a nutritionist, Craig and I had some tough curveballs thrown our way. I loved my job as a rock-climbing guide, but with the bad economy came bad news. Craig lost his job, which was our main source of income. Shortly after that happened, when I went for my yearly physical, I was a puddle. I cried at the drop of a hat, and I was worried that we were going to lose our house and our dream of adopting children.

My doctor immediately thought she would be a helpful "problem-solver" by offering me an antidepressant. She neither checked my vitamin D levels (which ended up being low after I had them checked with a new doctor) nor checked my liver health, which was also probably horrible with the high-carb diet I followed at the time. Also, I was training for a marathon, which added stress to my adrenal system. The doctor did not ask if I was taking a probiotic. Lastly, the doctor did not ask about my diet. (As you might remember from a previous story, this is the same doctor who didn't ask about my diet when I had severe IBS.) I believe doctors should ask about all these things before offering patients mind-altering and addictive drugs that have lots of side effects. We would save a heck of a lot of money on healthcare! Needless to say, after this visit, I changed doctors.

In biology class, we are taught that our blood is manufactured in the bone marrow. In traditional Chinese medicine, we are taught that our blood begins on the end of our fork. We really are what we eat.

CRAVING THE NUTRIENTS WE NEED

Before my passion for nutrition came along, I had a passion for donuts. I was an athlete and thought I could get away with eating whatever I wanted as long as I worked out. This was simply not true. Even though I ate enough calories, I was starving myself. Specifically, I was starving my brain. Even though my stomach was filled with "substance," my brain kept telling me to eat.

Our bodies are smart; they make us crave the nutrients we need. In my low-fat past, I always felt guilty about enjoying fatty foods. However, the human body is hardwired to crave cholesterol and fat because the body is made up of this crucial macronutrient, so don't feel guilty! You crave cholesterol and fat because they are critical to your health. When you eat real cholesterol and fat, you regulate insulin levels and trigger enzymes that convert food into energy.

liver, which increases the rate of depression. Following a keto-adapted, allergen-free diet increases serotonin without sacrificing your waistline.

LIVER FUNCTION AND DEPRESSION

Cholesterol from food controls your body's internal cholesterol production and protects your liver. Your liver governs how effectively your body burns fat and your mood. Some signs of a toxic liver are weight gain, depression, cellulite, abdominal bloating, indigestion, fatigue, mood swings, high blood pressure, elevated cholesterol, and skin rashes. Many people struggle with weight gain and a sluggish metabolism most of their lives, and they go through lots of unsuccessful yo-yo dieting. The reason these yo-yo diets fail is that they tackle the symptom rather than the cause. Weight gain is often the result of poor liver function. The liver performs more than 400 different jobs; it is the body's most important metabolism-enhancing organ. The liver acts as a filter to clear your body of toxins, metabolize protein, control hormonal balance, and enhance your immune system.

Your liver is a "worker bee" that can even regenerate its damaged cells. However, your liver is not invincible. When it is abused and lacks essential nutrients, or when it is overwhelmed by toxins and excess estrogens, it no longer performs as it should. Fat can build up in the liver and just under the skin, hormone imbalances can develop, and toxins increase and get into the bloodstream. The liver metabolizes fats, proteins, and carbohydrates for fuel. It breaks down amino acids from proteins into various components to help build muscle, which directly impacts your caloric burn. It also transports amino acids through the bloodstream for hormone balance, which is critical for avoiding water retention, bloating, cravings, and other undesirable weight issues. There are many different amino acids that have a variety of important jobs. For example, L-tryptophan is an amino acid that comes from protein that helps build serotonin.

The liver's most important function—and the one that puts it at greatest risk for damage—is to detoxify the numerous toxins that attack the body daily. A healthy liver detoxifies many damaging substances and eliminates them without polluting the bloodstream. Cleaning our livers and eating the right foods improves metabolism, and we start burning fat.

In traditional Chinese medicine, doctors first check the liver when a patient is depressed. A tired and toxic liver causes low thyroid function and depression. If you are depressed, we highly suggest having your liver enzymes checked. If they are elevated, use castor oil packs at least two or three times a week. Add a drop of dōTERRA Zendocrine oil (a combination of tangerine peel, rosemary leaf, geranium plant, juniper berry, and cilantro herb essential oils) to castor oil and rub it on the liver area. Cover the area with some wool flannel, a towel, and a hot water bottle. Let it sit for at least forty-five minutes. This works so miraculously, it is almost unbelievable.

Sadly, we work with many children with cancer who are going through chemo, which causes their livers to be very toxic. This castor-oil trick causes their liver enzymes to drop to normal levels.

LET COOKING BE THY MEDICINE

I work with clinics that specialize in treating depression. Many of them are connecting food with brain health. Let cooking be thy medicine! The other night, I made my Protein Noodle Lasagna from my book *Keto Restaurant Favorites.* As we gobbled it up, my son said, "Can I have another bowl? This is the best food ever!" Just hearing that made all the work of making it worthwhile. You don't get that sense of joy and fulfillment from reheating chicken nuggets or junky frozen food that's marketed to kids. Sure, it takes time to make healthy meals, but I find it totally worth it when I know I am feeding my family well!

> " Without a doubt, this has been the best way of eating I have found. I've been on virtually every diet out there, and Maria's way has been life-changing. So far, I've dropped three clothing sizes, feel so much better, and love that I don't have to count calories and keep records of food intake. I laugh at people who are mortified when they hear that I eat bacon and eggs every morning! I suffer no more constipation, no more IBS attacks, no more constant arthritic flare-ups or brain fog, no more depression, and no more lack of energy. Fibromyalgia? GONE! My medical doctor is totally on board with the keto-adapted way of life, and even my 82-year-old rheumatologist, whom I expected to cringe when I told him about this, totally approved and told me I was smart to make this choice!

—Laurie

CHOLESTEROL MEDICATION AND DEPRESSION

Have you been put on a statin drug to lower cholesterol as a "preventative measure"? If so, we suggest you find a new doctor! Not only are statins bad for your sex drive, muscle tissues, and memory, but they also exacerbate depression. The human brain is more than 60 percent fat. When we starve our brains and cells of valuable cholesterol, it has been proven to increase risk of depression by 300 percent![3]

Even though statin drugs cause a greater risk of a toxic liver, kidney failure, muscle damage, depression, and cataracts, they are still being pushed to the public as a "preventative measure"! Women are often mistakenly put on cholesterol-lowering drugs after menopause because cholesterol makes hormones. If your

FOOD AND MOOD

I had the great opportunity to be a speaker on a low-carb cruise to Alaska in 2017. I met some amazing people, including a woman named Amber. Amber is a carnivore food blogger with a unique story. Amber has bipolar disorder, but she no longer suffers from the symptoms or needs medication to manage it.

Food healed her. She eats only meat and eggs; that's it. If she gets carbs from vegetables or even certain spices, her illness comes back. Food is medicine!

Our brains are made up of more than 60 percent fat, so it makes sense that consuming fat helps regulate our moods.

ovaries are no longer producing these hormones, your cholesterol goes up in an effort to make your body produce the needed hormones. Many doctors place menopausal women on these drugs when trying to push cholesterol down. Men who take statins often have a lower sex drive or also take erectile dysfunction medication. You need cholesterol to make hormones.

MODIFICATIONS

Eat plenty of cholesterol. Low-fat, low-cholesterol diets can be very unhealthy, especially for women. Why? Cholesterol and saturated fat produce healthy hormones. All our major hormones are made from cholesterol—estrogen, progesterone, cortisol, DHEA, and testosterone. If you don't eat enough cholesterol, your body diverts it from your endocrine system to use for brain function and repair. When that happens, it's almost impossible for your body to maintain hormonal balance.

Stay away from all alcohol. Alcohol is a known depressant.

Get your hormones checked. Hormones influence neurotransmitter release and activity. If hormones are deficient or are off balance, neurotransmitters do not function well. Premenstrual syndrome (PMS) is a classic example of how low serotonin levels can temporarily shift each month. Mood, appetite, and sleep can be severely disrupted one to two weeks before the menstrual cycle. Another neurotransmitter, acetylcholine, decreases during menopause when dramatic changes in memory, mood, energy, sleep, weight, and sexual desire occur.

Get quality sleep. Lack of quality of sleep depresses mood. Many neurotransmitters responsible for proper sleep, especially serotonin, are produced during REM sleep around three to four hours after you have fallen asleep. Serotonin converts to melatonin, the sleep hormone. When serotonin levels are low, melatonin levels are also low. Disrupted sleep occurs, and fewer neurotransmitters are produced, which turns into a vicious cycle.

Re-evaluate your medications. Long-term use of acne medications, diet pills, stimulants, pain pills, narcotics, and recreational drugs can deplete neurotransmitter stores and damage your liver. Ma huang, Ephedra, and prescription diet pills use up large amounts of dopamine and serotonin.

Cut out neurotoxins. Cleaning agents, hair chemicals, pesticides, fertilizers, heavy metal toxicity, and recreational drugs cause harm to neurons and decrease neurotransmitter production. Excess caffeine, nicotine, and alcohol are neurotoxins. The overuse of the recreational drug Ecstasy drains serotonin and permanently damages the neurons.

Eat 100 percent gluten-free. After the digestive tract, the nervous system is the system that is most commonly affected by gluten. Gluten-free foods aren't necessarily the answer because they can inhibit healing and prevent you from getting off medication. Pre-packaged gluten-free foods often contain rice flour, which is higher in calories, higher in carbohydrates, and lower in nutrients than even regular flour. Rice flour can cause more inflammation, so our recommendation, of course, is to eat keto and avoid "gluten-free" packaged foods!

It is believed that gluten can cause depression in one of two ways:

- When you're sensitive to gluten, your immune system responds to the protein gliadin. Unfortunately, the protein gliadin is similar in structure to other proteins in the body, including those in the nerve and brain cells. A cross-reaction occurs when the immune system mistakes proteins in the body for gliadin. This cross-reaction is called cellular mimicry, and the outcome is that the body starts to attack its tissues that cause inflammation. When inflammation happens, a variety of issues can occur, including depression. Even if you do not experience digestive issues, gluten can still cause depression. You can have problems with gluten that show up in other parts of your body—not only the digestive tract. Gluten can attack any part of your body—joints, thyroid, gallbladder, nervous system, and cell membranes. It can cause a variety of serious problems, including multiple sclerosis. Even if you aren't having digestive issues, you still could have an allergy to gluten.

- Gluten also can interfere with protein absorption by causing an inability to absorb tryptophan (an amino acid in the brain), which is essential for brain health. Tryptophan is responsible for a feeling of well-being. A deficiency causes depression and anxiety. Ninety percent of serotonin production occurs in the digestive tract, so it makes sense that food influences your serotonin production, which can have a negative effect on your moods.

> " *I just want to tell everyone what a difference you've made in not only my family's life but my patients' lives, too. As a doctor, I was always pushing 'healthy whole grains' and fruits like bananas for potassium, but after looking at myself in the mirror, I knew something wasn't right with this idea of calories in and calories out. I was eating a very clean diet of 'healthy whole grains,' quinoa, and tons of fruit, but I was overweight, had adult acne, and was feeling a bit depressed. And I had anxiety when it came to food; counting points was not working for me.*
>
> *One of my patients gave me a copy of your book, and I was so inspired I decided to do a phone consult, which forever changed my life. I have to be honest, the first week was awful. I felt like one of my patients suffering from drug withdrawal, but now I understand that the sugars and grains were my drug. Your explanation on how the protein in the wheat is similar to other proteins in the body which was causing cellular mimicry in my nervous system and brain and was causing my slight depression made total sense. You taught me that I was gluten sensitive; this too was shocking to me since I didn't suffer from any intestinal issues. But after working with you for six weeks, I no longer felt depressed! Not only that, but I lost 31 pounds and no longer had to use my topical medication for adult acne (but after watching your cosmetics tutorial video, I realized how toxic those products were to my liver, which also contributed to my poor moods and inability to lose weight).*
>
> *You not only changed my life, but my kids are now 100% grain-free and enjoy picking out recipes from your kids' cookbook for snacks at school. I also feel so much better about setting a good example for my patients; I felt uncomfortable preaching to them about what to eat while being overweight. Now I know the whole truth, and I am forever grateful. The consult with you really changed my life more than you will ever realize.*

—Dr. Sally

Get more exercise. Exercise and movement help increase serotonin, too. Lifting weights and watching yourself in the mirror so you can see your strength gains can improve your serotonin levels. We have witnessed this with many clients!

Get outside. Get outside and enjoy nature.

Eliminate histamine-producing foods. Make sure to cut all histamine-producing foods, including strawberries, because high histamines block serotonin and can cause depression.

Add salt to food or drink homemade bone broth a few times a day. Doing so will help with energy and mood! When you first start your well-formulated low-carb lifestyle, you might notice that you get dizzy or feel faint when you stand up quickly; that means you are dehydrated! Just drinking water isn't going to work like it would with a high-carbohydrate diet. You need to add more salt! You can add more salt to your food, drink bone broth, or take sodium tablets. Salt is not the evil nutrient that we've been warned about. You must start thinking differently. Just as you've come to understand that eating more fat isn't harmful to your heart, you have to understand that a well-formulated ketogenic diet requires a lot more sodium. Dehydration causes depressed moods.

SUPPLEMENTS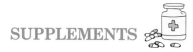

Bifidobacteria: Your mood comes from your gut. Having good gut bacteria increases serotonin. Take one capsule of *Bifidobacteria* daily.

SAMe: This nutrient transports molecules necessary to produce DNA and brain neurotransmitters. Take 400 milligrams of SAMe (it is best absorbed on an empty stomach), but do not take SAMe if you are taking an antidepressant.

Vitamin D: If you take vitamin D, always take 100 to 200 micrograms of vitamin K2. Take 1,000 IU per 25 pounds of your weight with a meal (it's fat-soluble) if you've had your levels tested and they're lower than 50.

D-HIST: High histamines block serotonin from being absorbed and often cause depression. D-HIST is a natural D-histamine, and you can find it at health food stores or online. If you have high histamine levels, add one capsule of D-HIST twice a day with food.

Getting Off Antidepressants

Getting off antidepressants is tough. Instead of taking antidepressants, you could consider natural alternatives, such as a high dose of vitamin D (making sure your level is above 45), *Bifidobacteria* (healthy bacteria has significant effects specifically on the feel-good neurotransmitter L-tryptophan), zinc, niacin, and magnesium. Also, drink lots of water, making sure to drink half of your body weight in ounces. (Hydrated cells are happy cells!) Before modifying your antidepressant regimen, though, you should always talk to your physician. A plan for weaning off the medication might look something like this: Halve or quarter your antidepressant for one week. At the start of the second week, take the half or quarter dose of your medication every other day. On the off days, take 400 milligrams of 5-HTP. Alternate between the reduced dose of your antidepressant and the 5-HTP for a week. At the beginning of the third week, under medical supervision, eliminate the prescription and take 400 milligrams of 5-HTP for a month along with 400 milligrams of SAMe. Continue taking 5-HTP and SAMe as needed.

Zinc: If you are an athlete and sweat a lot, you are likely low in zinc; the thyroid is a zinc hog. Being low in zinc can cause low thyroid, which results in low moods. Low zinc also can cause excess copper, which is the most common cause of postpartum depression. During pregnancy, copper levels increase significantly; after giving birth, the mother is unable to lower copper levels. Because zinc can cause upset stomach, start with 10 milligrams of zinc once a day for one week. Add 10 milligrams each week until you can take 50 milligrams per day without feeling nauseated.

Iodine: If you are using only a quality sea salt (which we recommend), you are not getting the iodine found in table salt. All our hormones need iodine to function. More than 80 percent of the U.S. population is deficient in iodine, which causes depression, lethargy, difficulty losing weight, dry skin, acne, hair loss, constipation, cold sensitivity in everyone, and poor brain development in children. We suggest taking 325 milligrams in the form of a kelp supplement once a day with food.

Gamma-linoleic acid (GLA): Gamma-linoleic acid and linoleic acid are essential for skin health, skin elasticity, and cellular structure. These fatty acids regulate hormones, including the thyroid and sex hormones. They improve nerve function and decrease pain caused by fibromyalgia, PMS, and migraine headaches. Women should take 1,500 milligrams of emu oil or 1,300 milligrams of evening primrose oil three times a day with meals. Men should take 600 milligrams of borage oil three times a day, preferably with food.

Potassium: Because you lose a lot of sodium through the diuretic effect of a low-carb diet, you eventually lose a lot of potassium, too. Keeping your potassium levels up helps to safeguard your lean muscle mass during weight loss. As with sodium, adequate potassium prevents cramping and fatigue. A deficiency in potassium causes low energy, heavy legs, salt cravings, and dizziness; you also might cry easily. Take 200 milligrams of potassium per day. Important: Do not take potassium if you are taking medication for high blood pressure.

EstroFactors: The liver is a filter of sorts. It detoxifies our bodies, protecting us from the harmful effects of chemicals, elements in food, environmental toxins, and even natural products of our metabolism, including excess estrogen. Anything that impairs liver function or ties up the detoxifying function will result in excess estrogen levels. EstroFactors are designed to detox excess bad estrogen. High estrogen levels can come from exposure to chemicals that mimic estrogen, such as many plastics (microwaving food in plastic dishes or using plastic wraps and containers) or eating non-organic food. People develop estrogen dominance because they eat a high-carb diet, consume excess fructose, drink alcohol, have a toxic liver, or are exposed to environmental factors such as pollution and topical chemicals. Take three capsules with food once a day for one month; then take one capsule daily for four more months.

Magnesium glycinate: Magnesium is a precursor to making serotonin. If you supplement magnesium, you need to take a very absorbable form of magnesium. We recommend 400 milligrams of magnesium glycinate when you wake because blood pressure is highest in the morning. (Do not use magnesium oxide or citrate because it will just cause loose stools.) We suggest taking 400 to 800 micrograms of magnesium glycinate at bedtime to help you relax and prepare for sleep.

5-HTP: This is an amino acid. The T stands for tryptophan, which increases serotonin. Tryptophan also helps with sleep quality. Add

200 to 400 milligrams, but do not take it if you're already taking an antidepressant. Note that for some people, L-tryptophan works better than 5-HTP. If 5-HTP doesn't work for you, try 1 to 5 grams of L-tryptophan.

FERTILITY AND PREGNANCY

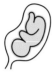

Estrogen, progesterone, cortisol, DHEA, and testosterone are made from cholesterol; if we don't eat enough, our bodies take cholesterol from our endocrine system to use for brain function and repair. When that happens, it's almost impossible for our bodies to maintain proper hormonal balance.

When women follow a low-fat diet, what do they eat instead? Carbohydrates! Those carbs are metabolized into sugars that cause weight gain and insulin resistance, which in turn disrupts ovulation because healthy estrogen is converted to androgens (testosterone). We see this classic sign of PCOS quite often. Starch, sugar, and caffeine increase the production of androgens, and women often complain about dark hairs on their face and inability to lose weight.

We cannot achieve proper hormonal balance and conceive babies without eating adequate amounts of saturated fat. Cholesterol is so important during fertility and pregnancy; it is the foundation of normal cell function, and it helps women digest fat-soluble vitamins like A, D, E, and K, which are essential for the formation of healthy fetuses. Full-fat dairy is filled with healthy cholesterol. People who are sensitive to dairy need to rely on other sources of saturated fats, such as coconut oil, quality animal fats, seafood, and egg yolks.

SATURATED FAT AND FERTILITY

Saturated fat and cholesterol make healthy hormones, including thyroid hormones, which also help with fertility. In June 2017, I had the opportunity to speak at Dr. Robert Kiltz's CNY Fertility Clinic in Syracuse, New York. His success rate for helping couples get pregnant is through the roof! Want to know his secret? He tells his clients to eat saturated fats—and lots of them! He is swamped with clients, and his prices are lower than any other fertility clinic's. He gets it! Diet comes first!

"

The ketogenic lifestyle is such a huge passion of mine—it has transformed my health and life as well as that of my family. I owe my life to this lifestyle. I had always been overweight, exhausted, and sick, even as a child. I tried literally everything to change my health and body, but nothing ever seemed to work. I was depressed, had thyroid issues, and eventually developed fertility problems, making it nearly impossible for my husband and me to have the children that we so desperately wanted. Fast-forward to several years of following the keto lifestyle, and my weight is under control for the first time in my life; I am joyful, energetic, and healthy. And, best of all, at the age of 30, the most recent 'side effect' is that we are due with our first child! Something I thought I would never get to experience! I'm getting a bit emotional writing this, but it has been the most magical health transformation I could have imagined. I literally owe every blessing in my life to the fact that I was fortunate enough to discover the keto diet, and I feel like it is my life's purpose to help others discover how to turn their lives around in the amazing way that I was able to. My only hope is that I can learn from those who went before me and paved the way with their passion for the same values as myself. I see what an impact you have made and continue to make in the lives and health of others, and it is such a beautiful thing that it moves me to tears. All I want in life is to leave a positive impact like that on the lives of my fellow humankind.

Thank you so much for your time and for all the good that you do in the world!

—Katelyn

POLYCYSTIC OVARIAN SYNDROME AND FERTILITY

Hormones are chemical messengers that activate numerous diverse processes in the body, including energy production. Often, one hormone signals the release of another hormone.

When a woman has polycystic ovarian syndrome (PCOS), her hormones fall out of balance. One hormone triggers another, which changes another, and sex hormones get out of whack.

In a healthy female body, the ovaries make a tiny amount of male sex hormones (androgens). In a woman with PCOS, her body starts making too many androgens, which often causes her

I never really talk about it because I am a very private person, but I didn't have a period until I was sixteen. All my friends would talk about it, and I just acted as though I didn't like having a period. However, I knew I was different.

Once I got my first period, the second one didn't come as soon as it should have, and they were very sporadic and painful. I had dark facial hair and was on antibiotics for excessive acne. These are all classic signs of PCOS.

Even when I started to diet and lose weight, I was doing it the wrong way, and my PCOS wasn't going away. I lived on cereal and skim milk, carrots dipped in mustard (gross, I know!), and salads with fat-free French dressing. I ate sugar, sugar, and more sugar!

As I studied nutrition in college, I started to eat lower-carb, which helped me in many ways. However, I didn't start to heal until I added more saturated fat (yes, I said "saturated fat") and cholesterol.

Don't wait so long to seek help like I did. I suffered quietly, but you don't have to suffer through this alone! If you suffer from PCOS, act now to get on the path to feeling better.

I believe that everything happens for a reason—even bad things such as PCOS. My past brought me to my future. I have a wonderful job in which I can help educate you about the truth! But more than anything, my past led me to my two precious boys.

to stop ovulating, grow excessive facial and body hair, and develop acne. Caffeine aggravates and increases androgens, so you should eliminate caffeine from your diet.

A woman with PCOS has too much insulin and is insulin resistant. When her body doesn't use insulin well, her blood sugar goes up. Over time, this increases her risk of diabetes.

As you know by now, too much insulin is caused by carbohydrates and sugar, and cholesterol is what makes healthy hormones. We know this from studying breast-fed babies. Breast milk is primarily made up of cholesterol, which is essential for the baby to develop gonads, a thyroid, and other hormones. We get so frustrated when we hear dietitians recommend cutting all cholesterol and saturated fats. If cholesterol is so important to babies, at what point in a person's life does it change from being a crucial nutrient to a demonized nutrient?

Cholesterol is so important to the human body that nature has devised a backup plan in the event your diet falls short. When that happens, your liver steps in to make cholesterol to give your body a baseline level. If your liver gets overused and tired, thyroid issues also develop because the thyroid hormone T4 is converted into the activated T3 hormone in your liver, not in your thyroid! Taking care of your liver is extra important!

In a short six-month period, a ketogenic diet for PCOS leads to significant reductions in weight as well as lower testosterone, LH/FSH (luteinizing hormone and follicle-stimulating hormone) ratio, and fasting serum insulin in women with PCOS. All three of these things help reverse PCOS. It might take time to heal decades of abusing your cells, but you will heal.

Estrogen dominance is a huge factor of PCOS. Alcohol is a huge estrogenic toxin (see page 66). Another thing that causes estrogen dominance is topical chemicals and makeup. In the Healthy and Environmental Research on Makeup of Salinas Adolescents (HERMOSA) study in 2016, researchers found that when participants changed their toxic makeup for only three days, the levels of chemicals in their urine went down by 45 percent![4]

You might read that someone with PCOS needs to eliminate red meat. What these studies don't tell you is that they use conventional meat filled with hormones. Please avoid that. Hormones in food are not a good idea for anyone, but especially those who already have hormonal imbalances. Primitive people gave the prized red meat and organ meat to the fertile tribesmen and women to ensure the survival of the tribe. They knew that to have a healthy reproduction, the men and women needed quality protein and fats, and that hasn't changed over time.

The following factors can increase PCOS and/or hormonal imbalances:

- Alcohol
- Caffeine
- Carbs and sugar
- Hormones in foods like non-organic meats, flax, chia, and soy
- Trans fats (they form a crust around cells that increases insulin resistance)
- Topical products and other obesogens (foreign chemical compounds that disrupt normal development and balance of lipid metabolism)
- Lack of cholesterol consumption
- Excessive stress

NOTE

You don't have to be overweight to have PCOS or diabetes. I've had numerous clients with type 2 diabetes who were underweight. The keto diet isn't just about weight loss. You can and will gain weight if you eat too many calories, even if you are in ketosis.

Certain supplements can also increase healing time by saturating the cells with therapeutic doses of needed nutrients.

MODIFICATIONS

For fertility and a healthy pregnancy, do not limit fat; instead, add a lot of saturated fat. Cut all dairy from your diet, however, because a sensitivity to dairy can cause an inability to carry to term and can lead to miscarriage.

SUPPLEMENTS

Iodine: All our hormones need iodine to function, which is why table salt is fortified with it. However, if you are using a quality sea salt, you need to know that it is devoid of iodine, which is why we suggest supplementing with iodine (or eating oysters, which also are filled with zinc, daily). More than 80 percent of the U.S. population is deficient in iodine, leading to miscarriages, lethargy, dry skin, hair loss, constipation, and poor brain development in babies.

Selenium: Selenium is essential for the conversion of T4 to T3, which is the active form of thyroid hormone. During pregnancy, the immune system goes into overdrive to protect the fetus. After delivering the baby, the mother often produces antibodies against her thyroid; which is one reason women suffer autoimmune thyroid more than men. Adding selenium while pregnant is not only very safe but it also lowers the autoimmune response after giving birth. Take 200 micrograms daily with or without food.

Bifidobacteria: The first two years of life are crucial for long-term immune responses. A pregnant and breastfeeding mother taking probiotics promotes health in infants. Probiotics prevent eczema, diarrhea, diaper rash, and cradle cap; lower the baby's chances of developing food allergies; and eliminate thrush. Take one capsule of *Bifidobacteria* daily with a teaspoon of coconut vinegar.

There are other supplements that help with fertility, but they need to be determined by each individual's needs. It requires an analysis of the body's symptoms and areas of deficiency.

> ### TIP
> During a vaginal birth, the baby is coated in a mucus filled with healthy microbes that give the baby good gut bacteria for a lifetime.

MENOPAUSE: WEIGHT GAIN AND OSTEOPENIA

One of the most frustrating things we deal with when women enter menopause is the overwhelming number of doctors who put these women on statins to combat high cholesterol. We can't stress this enough: Cholesterol makes *healthy hormones*!

During menopause, progesterone and the healthy estrogen from your ovaries (remember there are three types of estrogen) are declining rapidly. Your cholesterol starts to increase to try to make your ovaries produce progesterone and healthy estrogen. However, the ovaries aren't responding, which results in high cholesterol, and doctors see this increased cholesterol as being bad.

A well-formulated keto diet works for menopausal symptoms by replacing glucose that's lacking from the hormone-deprived brain. When glucose can't get into the brain because of insulin resistance, it causes hot flashes and low cognitive function— two common complaints of our clients who are going through menopause. Ketone bodies are water-soluble fat that can pinch hit for glucose in the brain and other tissues.

❝ _____

Hi Maria! You have been so helpful to me [as I've gone] through menopause. I have been following your blog in its various iterations for about five years. I'm 54, healthy, fit, I don't take any prescriptions, and I've never had a weight problem. When perimenopause hit a few years ago, I put on too many pounds. Nothing I would do would take the menopause pounds back off. When I hit around 20 pounds over my normal and the new slacks were getting too tight, I consulted with you and followed your meal plans. In a month, all of the menopause weight was off and I felt like me again. It's staying off!

I no longer crave sugar. I don't have many cravings for 'crunchy-salty,' but I have keto-friendly options for that. I'm learning to cook a new way, to shop for food a new way, and to even eat out a new way. Oh, and OMG, fat bombs!

My pantry looks a LOT different today than it used to . . . and I like it.

Thank you. _____

—Tracy

When your brain is deprived of healthy hormones after decades of exposure, you start to experience hot flashes. Estrogen is closely involved in the transportation of glucose into the brain cells. When we are menstruating and have healthy hormones, estrogen transports about 40 percent more glucose into the brain cells than would be shuttled there without progesterone and healthy estrogen. When the progesterone and healthy estrogen goes away at menopause, the transportation of glucose into the brain cells decreases, and the brain cells become a little starved for energy. The hypothalamus responds to this starvation by increasing the release of norepinephrine (adrenaline), which increases the level of sugar in the blood to raise the heart rate. The increased heart rate causes an increase in the body temperature. A hot flash is an outward sign that the brain is trying to protect itself from blood sugar starvation.

During menopause, bone loss also occurs. Progesterone builds healthy bones in women, so as the level of progesterone declines, bone loss results. We see a lot of menopausal clients whose bone density scans show that they are suffering from osteopenia and osteoporosis (see "Bone Health" on page 162).

Ultimately, you want to use fat instead of carbs to fuel your body. Carbohydrates promote inflammation and lead to hormonal imbalances that further intensify symptoms. Women who are already in menopause and halt the detrimental symptoms with a well-formulated keto diet often see a regular menstrual cycle return, a reduction in belly fat tissue, and increased libido.

MODIFICATIONS

Eat keto! Getting quality fats and cholesterol helps increase hormone production.

SUPPLEMENTS

Evening primrose oil or emu oil: The fatty acids in evening primrose oil help regulate hormones (including the thyroid) and improve nerve function. Take 1,300 milligrams three times daily. Or take 1,500 milligrams of emu oil three times a day with food.

EstroFactors: EstroFactors is designed to detox excess bad estrogen. Supplement with three capsules with food once a day for one month, and then take one capsule daily for four more months.

L-carnitine: L-carnitine is an amino acid that aids in the breakdown of calories by shuttling fatty acids into the mitochondria, which are the fat-burning powerhouses in our cells. First thing after waking, take 3 grams of L-carnitine to increase energy, increase weight loss and focus, and lower triglycerides.

CoQ10: Take 400 milligrams for mitochondria building, especially if you have ever taken a cholesterol-lowering drug.

Choline: Most women are predisposed to an acetylcholine deficiency, which often increases with perimenopause. Estrogen and testosterone stimulate the production of acetylcholine. As those hormones decline, so does the production of this essential brain chemical; the result is symptoms such as memory loss, dry skin, and weight gain. Egg yolks are filled with choline! Bring on the hollandaise sauce! Take 500 milligrams of a choline supplement twice a day with food.

Pro-Gest cream: Pro-Gest cream includes a wild yam extract that helps with sleep and lowers anxiety as well as hormonal migraines. If you wake up too early in the morning and have poor sleep, use ¼ to ½ teaspoon of natural Pro-Gest cream each night. We suggest a cream without additives. You can find Pro-Gest cream online or at a natural health store.

I USE PRO-GEST

Because I grew up with PCOS, I use Pro-Gest cream every night or I can't sleep. It has been a godsend!

ALZHEIMER'S DISEASE AND DEMENTIA

Inflammation causes you to have a large waistline and starts the snowball effect of memory loss and Alzheimer's disease. Sadly, we are watching Maria's grandmother go through this right now. She is an amazingly strong woman who decided to get her doctorate degree in her sixties after her husband died. She has always been brilliant and loves to teach kids to read, so she went back to school to learn more so she could pass on her knowledge. She could have traveled the world, but instead she taught kids. The sad part is that by the time she received her PhD, her memory had already started to decline.

Alzheimer's disease is often referred to as type 3 diabetes. It is a metabolic syndrome of the brain. Insulin resistance is a precursor to Alzheimer's disease. When Alzheimer's sets in, the brain can

LOW CHOLESTEROL CAN LEAD TO ALZHEIMER'S DISEASE

Twenty-five percent of the body's cholesterol is in the brain, and a deficiency in cholesterol can lead to Alzheimer's disease.

no longer use glucose for energy, so it must use a different source. Enter ketones! Adding medium-chain triglycerides (MCT) in high doses multiple times a day, along with a keto diet, helps patients who suffer from memory loss.

Glycation is when glucose binds to proteins. This process produces free radicals and inflammation, which are markers of Alzheimer's disease. Determining whether your body is in glycation is simple; you examine your A1c level. If your hemoglobin A1c is high, the free radicals in your body are greatly increased. Studies show that high hemoglobin A1c levels are a marker for the progression of atrophy of the brain.

Ketones aren't just fuel for our bodies; they are also great for brain health. They provide substrates to help repair damaged neurons and membranes, which is why we push a high-fat and low-carb diet for clients who suffer from Alzheimer's disease and seizures.

Ketones are non-glycating, which means that they don't have a caramelizing aging effect on the body. The mitochondria are the energy-producing factories of our cells. They work much better on a ketogenic diet because they can increase energy levels in an unwavering, long-lasting, and efficient way.

A ketogenic diet also increases the energetic output of our mitochondria because these amazing "powerhouse" factories of our cells are essentially designed to use fat as energy. When we

66 —————————————————

My 90-year-old mother has had dementia for ten years, and her cognition is improving now that she is in ketosis most of the time. I spent last week training all of her in-home caregivers on probiotic, mineral supplementation, and water needs.

I also eliminated the last few sources of sugar (bananas, applesauce, rice) and replaced [them] with more fat that she can tolerate. This week she is more mobile, conversational, and alert! All of the caregivers have been texting me stating what improvements they are seeing. I've been a little nervous experimenting on my mom, but you have given me the knowledge and confidence to do so. Wish I had had this info before my dad passed as I think he would have benefited greatly.

—Gail

switch from using glucose to using fat in the mitochondria, the following things happen:

- The burden on the mitochondria is reduced.
- The manifestation of energy-producing genes is improved.
- The output is increased.
- The load of inflammatory by-products is decreased.

Glucose needs to be processed first in the cell before it can be passed into the mitochondria. Energy sources from fat don't need this processing; they go straight into the mitochondria for energy.

MODIFICATIONS

Add 1 tablespoon of coconut oil to each meal or eat fat bombs three to six times a day.

Use coconut oil or MCT oil in your cooking and salad dressings whenever possible.

SUPPLEMENTS

Acetyl-L-carnitine: This is an amino acid from protein that's used for brain-related issues, such as Alzheimer's disease, memory, depression, and brain-related Lyme disease. Right after waking, take 3 grams of acetyl-L-carnitine.

Magnesium L-threonate: This very absorbable form of magnesium is especially good for brain function, memory, cognition, and Alzheimer's disease. Take 400 milligrams right after waking and right before bedtime.

CoQ10: Mitochondria are the "powerhouses" of cells that help with cognition. Take 400 milligrams of CoQ10 with food for mitochondria building.

Gamma-linoleic acid (GLA): Gamma-linoleic acid is essential for skin health, skin elasticity, and cellular structure. These fatty acids regulate hormones, including thyroid and sex hormones. They also improve nerve function and cognition. Women should take 1,500 milligrams of emu oil or 1,300 milligrams of evening primrose oil three times a day with food. Men should take 600 milligrams of borage oil three times a day with food.

Zinc: Zinc is essential for creating DNA, a healthy immune system, building proteins, and triggering enzymes. It also helps cells communicate by functioning as a neurotransmitter. Zinc can cause nausea, so start with 10 milligrams a day for one week and then increase by 10 milligrams each week until you can take 50 milligrams in one dose without feeling nauseated.

Vitamin B12: Low B12 causes severe memory issues. Take one capsule of vitamin B12 (2,000 milligrams) daily.

Choline: Most women are predisposed to acetylcholine deficiency, which often sets in with perimenopause. Estrogen and testosterone stimulate the production of acetylcholine. As those hormones decline, so does the production of this essential brain chemical; the result is symptoms like memory loss, dry skin, and weight gain. Egg yolks are filled with choline, too, so bring on the hollandaise! Take 500 milligrams daily.

Ketone supplements: Ketone supplements increase blood ketone levels and can help provide more fuel to the brain. Research on ketone supplements is underway and has started to show some good results.

BONE HEALTH (OSTEOPENIA AND OSTEOPOROSIS)

Let's start by covering a few facts about bones and calcium.

You might not realize that the cellular wall of bone is made up of fat. And it's not just any fat; those cellular walls of your bones are mainly made up of saturated fat! Yes, if you only use olive oil and avoid saturated fats—like your doctor might recommend for

MY AMAZING GREAT-GRANDMOTHER

When I was seven years old, we were at a family gathering at my grandparents' house for Christmas. My ninety-year-old great-grandma, Minnie Kress, who was a whipper-snapper, was at the party. She was an amazing and strong woman who was never afraid of butter or lard. She mistakenly went through the basement door (instead of the bathroom door) and tumbled all the way down the steps onto a concrete floor, and she did not break one bone! Given her age, I can't believe that fall didn't shatter her bones. I suspect that her diet high in saturated fat helped her have strong bones.

heart health (terrible advice)—you are putting your bones at risk.

Bones are alive and are either breaking down (osteoclasts) or building up (osteoblasts). Females build 42 percent of their bone mass between the ages of twelve and eighteen, so you need to watch what your teens are eating and drinking. Sodas and sports drinks ruin the strength of bones. Give your kids quality sources of calcium instead.

Bones also need collagen. Our favorite way to give them collagen is bone broth. Bone broth is awesome for supplying collagen, and it's high in well-absorbed minerals.

Antacids increase the risk of hip fractures. Chewable antacids are made from calcium carbonate, which is a terrible form of calcium. One study found that antacid pills increase fracture risk by 44 percent![5] European doctors prescribe antacids for a maximum of two weeks, which is what the manufacturers' dosing instructions (in both Europe and the United States) clearly state. Doctors in the U.S. write more than 100 million antacid prescriptions each year, and many of those prescriptions are for babies. This is in addition to over-the-counter antacid use.

If you have low hydrochloric acid, you can't absorb the vitamins and minerals needed for proper bone health. Consequently, this is another place where antacids can cause a problem. If you have been on acid blockers or have a thyroid issue, you likely are deficient in hydrochloric acid. Our bodies also produce less hydrochloric acid as we age. You can do everything right with your diet, but you will not benefit from those nutrients if you can't absorb them! People with celiac disease can't absorb nutrients for healthy bones.

Six years ago I was told I have osteopenia, the beginning stages of osteoporosis. I started using almond flour and added magnesium six months ago. Last week I had a bone density test, and my results were astonishing! In fact, the nurse was stunned. My hip area increased 8.7 percent, and my spine increased 1.2 percent! She told me most women lose 1 percent per year while going through menopause. Thank you, Maria, for all your knowledge. I just received your Sweets cookbook and will be purchasing your slow cooker and one other to complete my collection! Love your blog and all the information!

—Kim

TIP

In our opinion, the most important bone-building supplement is vitamin K2, which is found in organ meat. How often do *you* eat organ meat? Yep, that's what we thought. We don't eat a lot of organ meat, either, so we give our kids K2 supplements. We also hide ground-up liver in our chili and lasagna.

Magnesium deficiency is a common cause of calcium not getting into bones. However, you shouldn't waste your money on calcium-magnesium supplements. Calcium and magnesium are "frenemies," or friends that compete for the same resources, and thus you shouldn't take them together. We do not recommend calcium supplements. However, a quality magnesium supplement, such as the magnesium glycinate form, is a good idea. We used to get magnesium from the water supply, but today we get much of our water from bottles and other filtered sources. Without adequate magnesium and vitamin K2 (see below), calcium is deposited in areas it shouldn't be, causing kidney stones and plaque buildup on teeth and in arteries. Taking a quality magnesium supplement at night (start with 400 milligrams) will help calm you down and help you sleep. Halibut is also high in magnesium.

BONE LOSS

Everyone seems to want a faster thyroid (lower TSH), but that is not healthy. A faster thyroid leads to bone loss because your body can't absorb nutrients. If your thyroid works too quickly, you can suffer from many issues, including sleeplessness, diarrhea, hunger, and anxiety, because everything is going too fast.

Low progesterone causes bone loss. You don't need to be in menopause to be low in progesterone. If you find yourself waking up at 2 or 3 a.m. and you aren't able to get back to sleep, or if you have high anxiety, we suggest you get your progesterone checked. Maria loves Pro-Gest all-natural cream by Emerita, which you can find at health food stores and online.

Progesterone Increases Bone Growth

Estrogen's role in osteoporosis is only a minor one. Estrogen replacement therapy reduced bone breakdown, but only progesterone can increase new bone growth. Progesterone deficiency results in bone loss. In a three-year study of sixty-three postmenopausal women with osteoporosis, women who used a topical progesterone cream experienced an average increase in bone mass density of 8 percent in the first year, 5 percent in the second year, and 4 percent in the third year. Untreated women in this age category typically lose 1.5 percent of their bone mass density per year. The use of natural progesterone along with dietary and lifestyle changes can stop—and possibly reverse—osteoporosis, regardless of your age.

Low vitamin D is a common cause of bone loss. Is your level not rising? You must get sunlight without the filter of sunscreen. You need UV light to activate cholesterol phosphates. How much vitamin D do you need? Well, if you are in the sun without sunscreen, you make about 20,000 to 30,000 IU per hour. That means you get 5,000 to 7,500 IU in fifteen minutes! Get a blood test to determine your vitamin D level, and if it is below 45, add a supplement or get more natural sun exposure. If you are taking a vitamin D supplement, you must take it with food because it is fat soluble. We also recommend taking vitamin D in the morning because it increases serotonin and lowers melatonin (supporting the body's natural circadian rhythm). If you take vitamin D before bed, it can cause sleep issues. You need 1,000 IU per 25 pounds of body weight.

To help prevent bone loss, stay away from these bone robbers:

- **Sugar:** Sugar can rob minerals from bones, which is why active kids shouldn't eat that junk, either!

- **Prescription drugs designed to slow bone loss:** Some prescription drugs that are intended to prevent bone loss actually make bones even harder and more brittle![6] They basically kill the bones. If someone who is on these drugs takes a bad fall, his or her bones might shatter rather than break because they are so hard and brittle.

- **Trans fat and alcohol:** Both these things can contribute to the weakening of bones.

GLUCOSE BURNING VERSUS KETONE BURNING

Your health and lifespan will be determined by which fuel source you use for energy. What you decide to put into your mouth affects every hormone in your body, including insulin, leptin, ghrelin, and human growth hormone. Those nutrients tell your cells what to do. If you choose glucose as your fuel source, you are going to crave glucose. And you are going to crave a lot of glucose because your body can't store much for anaerobic emergencies. We have glucose around because it can be burned without oxygen. Everyone stores a little in case of an emergency, but we couldn't survive on burning glucose alone.

Our largest source of glucose is protein—in other words, our muscles and bones—which is a huge problem!

If you are addicted to glucose and your hormones are telling your cells to burn glucose, you get cravings for carbs to fuel that addiction. Those carbs raise your insulin levels, which leads to insulin resistance as well as the formation of more fat made from that glucose. Even more disturbing is what happens while you sleep. If you are a sugar burner, you still need to burn glucose while you are sleeping. Because you are not consuming glucose during sleep, your body gets that glucose by tearing down your lean mass and bones, leading to muscle and bone loss. The biggest cause of osteoporosis has nothing to do with calcium. Instead, the main cause is the body breaking down bones during sleep to feed a glucose addiction.

The only way to burn fat as your primary fuel is to teach your body—and, more importantly, your hormones—to dig into your fat stores for energy. Doing so improves your insulin and leptin sensitivity and ultimately allows your body to stop robbing you of bone and muscle mass.

MODIFICATIONS

Ketogenic eating helps build healthy bones in many ways:
- The keto diet is high in healthy saturated fats that our bodies use to make the cell walls of our bones.
- Cholesterol in foods makes healthy hormones (especially progesterone, the thyroid hormone).
- The keto diet is free of sugar, which is the main bone robber.
- The keto diet is free of gluten and trans fat, two other bone robbers.

We recommend strength training for strong and healthy bones. Strength training is great for increasing bone density.

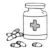

SUPPLEMENTS

Vitamin D: Take 1,000 IU per 25 pounds you weigh if your vitamin D level is less than 45. Read more about vitamin D in the "High Blood Pressure" section (pages 123 to 125).

Vitamin K2: This vitamin helps get calcium into your bones. Take 200 micrograms daily.

Hydrochloric acid (HCl): HCl helps with the absorption of minerals. Take one or two capsules (500 to 600 milligrams) with each meal.

Magnesium glycinate: This quality form of magnesium is easily absorbable and helps with bone building. Take 400 to 800 milligrams daily.

Pro-Gest cream: Low progesterone is the most common cause of bone loss of women. Women should use ½ teaspoon of Pro-Gest cream per day.

AUTOIMMUNE DISEASE

"

I know you get a lot of messages from clients—but I wanted to tell you about something exciting happening in my little cul-de-sac! I first started following your blog and purchasing your cookbooks in late 2012. At that time, I'd been hospitalized several times for ulcerative colitis, weighed about 90 pounds, and had developed allergies to the medications commonly used to treat the autoimmune condition. I had been put on Remicade—a very strong biologic drug that suppresses the immune system—just to keep my body from destroying itself further. Well, long story short, I used food to heal myself. In the past three years, I've gone from being barely able to get out of bed, in and out of the hospital and having to take strong cancer-causing drugs, to thriving, being able to run and lift weights and being off all dangerous medications! Believe it or not, that's not the exciting part. My family and neighbors have watched this transformation, and just this week, two of them have approached me about what I eat and how it has helped heal me. I directed them to your site, and they each purchased several cookbooks (your husband actually sent one of them a book that was no longer available on Amazon). They started their journey into healthy ketogenic foods this morning. Just wanted to let you know [that] being healthy and being excited about it is contagious! Thanks for all your help.

—Mica

There are numerous differences between food allergies and full-blown autoimmune disorders. The immune system's job is to free the body of foreign substances, such as viruses and bacteria, that might damage it. The immune system also builds protection against these invaders in case they try to attack again. This process is referred to as the immune response. However, the immune response can react incorrectly to normal body tissues. If the immune system believes that a part of the body is a foreign substance, it will attack those tissues—a process called an autoimmune response, which occurs in autoimmune disorders such as Hashimoto's thyroiditis, Graves' disease, celiac disease, rheumatoid arthritis, multiple sclerosis, and lupus. Problems arise when the body overreacts so aggressively that it creates an allergic reaction; the foreign element that triggers the allergic reaction is considered an allergen.

For example, celiac disease is an autoimmune disorder triggered by the ingestion of gluten. Gluten stimulates the production of immunoglobulins that attack the villi lining the small intestine. Celiac disease is often mistakenly thought of an allergic illness because, like an allergy, it requires a foreign substance to generate it. Celiac disease is not a wheat allergy, nor is it a gluten allergy. Many cases of celiac disease are asymptomatic; the gut morphological changes may be minimal, so it cannot be recognized.[7] Untreated celiac disease causes the activation of a type of white blood cell called a T lymphocyte (or T cell), along with other parts of the immune system; this activation increases the risk of gastrointestinal lymphomas. A wheat allergy, on the other hand, would not cause any of these problems.

Another difference between autoimmune conditions and allergies is that autoimmune conditions persist for life, while allergies can sometimes be outgrown.[8] If caught early enough—and if you eliminate 100 percent of the gluten from your diet—you can eliminate the other autoimmune disorders that you might be suffering from because of celiac disease.[9]

Celiac disease is characterized by the presence of antibodies, which is why we always send our clients to get a full-panel thyroid test with antibodies, a test that is not typically run unless you ask (beg) for it to be run. These antibodies are antigliadin, anti-endomysium, and anti-reticulin.

The incidence of celiac disease in people with autoimmune disorders has been shown to be increasing up to thirty-fold as compared to the general population. Often, celiac disease occurs without symptoms. The identification of "silent celiac" is imperative because celiac disease has been found to be the gateway disorder to other autoimmune conditions, including autoimmune thyroid disorders (Hashimoto's thyroiditis or Graves' disease) and type 1 diabetes.

We're often asked why celiac disease occurs in some people. There is confusion about what really causes this disease. One theory is that celiac disease is triggered after an infection by a type of virus that biologically resembles gluten. After the infection, the body can no longer differentiate between the invading virus and gluten, which causes the body to react by releasing mucus into the intestinal tract upon gluten exposure and causing damage to the intestines. This is considered "molecular mimicry." It's important to understand that even if the bacteria or virus triggering the attack is removed, the autoimmunity never turns off. The body continues to produce antibodies and attack healthy tissue even though the primary trigger is gone.

Molecular mimicry has been shown to launch a snowball effect of autoimmune responses. The theory is that molecular mimicry is the result of autoimmune disease, not a cause of the autoimmunity, which tells us that molecular mimicry is definitely a factor in the progression of preexisting conditions that trigger autoimmune disease. However, because we know that molecular mimicry is the result of autoimmune disease, we know that something else is responsible for triggering it in the first place.

With celiac disease, gluten (a non-self antigen) finds its way inside the body and causes a cross-reaction. When the body develops an allergy to gluten, it creates antibodies that remember gluten's structure. If you eat gluten-containing grains, those antibodies set off an inflammatory response. But other foods have a protein similar in structure to gluten and can also cause an inflammatory response. However, this evolution in thinking shows this cross-reaction to be only an effect of other preexisting conditions.[10] This is notable because, in order to heal, we need to discover what else is confusing the immune system. It is disturbing to find that 60 percent of adults never completely heal from celiac disease despite following a gluten-free diet.[11] Another study found that only 8 percent of adult patients with celiac disease eating a gluten-free diet reached "normalization," in which their intestines completely recovered.[12]

However, there is new research that might help people with celiac for good. Researcher and physician Alessio Fasano has been on the leading edge of autoimmune and celiac disease exploration. In 2011, he published a paper titled "Leaky Gut and Autoimmune Diseases," which presented a new theory suggesting prevention and reversal of autoimmune disease are possible.

Fasano finds that autoimmune responses occur for three reasons:

- There is an exposure to an environmental trigger. In other words, gluten = celiac disease.
- There is a genetic predisposition to autoimmunity. In other words, HLA DQ2 and DQ8 are genes that can make you more likely to develop celiac disease.
- Leaky gut (also known as increased intestinal permeability) could be the culprit.[13]

Using this knowledge, we can develop a plan to heal from celiac disease. We need to not only get rid of the trigger (gluten) but also resolve the leaky gut. That means we need to heal the gut tissue and restore both the proper intestinal permeability (allowing the passage of good material through the intestinal wall while blocking the bad) and the fingerlike villi in the intestines in order to function fully again. Gut permeability is also promoted by things like antibiotic use and chlorinated water.

Fasano's study tells us that if you have celiac disease, you also have leaky gut. Leaky gut causes other proteins found in foods to leak into your bloodstream, which is detrimental because your blood doesn't recognize this foreign substance and attacks it, causing the autoimmune response to continue. In some cases, this necessitates the elimination of other common allergens, such as dairy and eggs (which we usually love on low-carb diets), because those might be causing an autoimmune response, too.

MODIFICATIONS

Cut all dairy and gluten, which are the most common allergens that cause autoimmune responses.

SUPPLEMENTS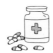

Bifidobacteria: Seventy percent of your immunity comes from your gut. Keep it healthy with probiotics. Take one capsule daily with a tablespoon of coconut vinegar or a can of sardines for prebiotics.

Glutathione: Glutathione is a super-antioxidant for cellular health. Take 500 milligrams with each meal.

CoQ10: CoQ10 aids in mitochondria building. Take 400 milligrams with your first meal of the day.

Alpha-lipoic acid (ALA): ALA is a neuroprotective antioxidant that can cross the blood-brain barrier (a highly selective membrane that separates circulating blood from the brain). It is also great for reducing inflammation, is fantastic as a heavy metal chelator (that is, it detoxes harmful heavy metals), and helps with insulin sensitivity. Take 400 milligrams once daily with food. Make sure it comes from a German source; Chinese sources often contain harmful additives.

Zinc: Zinc is essential for creating DNA, promoting a healthy immune system, building proteins, and triggering enzymes. It also helps cells communicate by functioning as a neurotransmitter. As previously noted, zinc can cause nausea, so start with 10 milligrams once a day with food. Do this for one week. Each week, add another 10 milligrams. By week five, you should be able to take 50 milligrams with a meal without becoming nauseated.

Vitamin D: Take 1,000 IU per 25 pounds of body weight if your level is less than 45. Read more about vitamin D in the "High Blood Pressure" section (pages 123 to 125).

CHRONIC PAIN AND INFLAMMATION (ARTHRITIS, FIBROMYALGIA)

Our hearts go out to all the people suffering from fibromyalgia and chronic fatigue syndrome. These are debilitating diseases that doctors often dismiss. We, however, believe that there are many causes, and our clients who follow our meal plans and supplement

"

Hi, Maria. You have been helping me get my life back by getting healthy. My main request was to help me get pregnant. Since starting your way less than three months ago, I have lost 31 pounds and am off all my autoimmune disease medications. And today, I can tell you that I found out I am expecting. I am only a few weeks along, and so I can't share with everyone yet, but I owe you my gratitude. After a year-long emotional journey, your way restored my body back to health.

—Carrie

regimes have had much success. Fibromyalgia is a disorder characterized by soft tissue pain and fatigue, which is made worse because the pain makes it difficult for fibromyalgia sufferers to sleep.

Vasoactive neuropeptides (protein-like substances that influence inflammatory control mechanisms) play a huge role in fibromyalgia and chronic fatigue syndrome. In a healthy body, these neuropeptides are eagerly catalyzed to small peptide fragments that activate hormones, neurotransmitters, and the immune system. These neuropeptides, along with their binding sites, are immunogenic and are known to be related to a wide variety of autoimmune diseases. Neuropeptides play an essential role in sustaining vascular flow (blood flow) in our organs, controlling memory and attentiveness, and controlling thermoregulation. They are powerful immune regulators with powerful anti-inflammatory activity, and they play a significant role in protecting the nervous system. When this neuropeptide is malfunctioning, pain and other detrimental issues start to snowball.

Vasoactive neuropeptides are also cotransmitters for acetylcholine.

At the age of 62, I was told to quit working. I had been taking eight high-powered meds daily. Those pills barely masked the pain from an inoperable situation. My exhausted, painful body was carrying over 40 pounds of extra weight. I was a mess. I struggled to work at a job I loved. As a cashier, I was able to see friends. Even though I didn't go out after work because of pain, at least I could see people during the day. Reluctantly, I quit my job. My mind wasn't ready to retire, but my body was.

At the age of 65, I found Maria. It's been over nine months since I started following her. After all this time, I still find improvements in my life. The most recent incident happened when I volunteered at a school book fair. Friends said they hadn't seen me in quite a while. At least they thought they hadn't. What was really happening was that they did not recognize me. It has been wonderful to hear all the compliments on how I look. Everyone was happy to see that I was no longer using a walker or a cane.

It is exciting to think of how much better I will be in another nine months!

—Pam

MODIFICATIONS

Let's dive into why a well-formulated keto diet helps reduce the debilitating side effects of fibromyalgia and chronic fatigue:

- **Inflammation:** One reason so many people are dealing with inflammation is a rapid rise in blood sugar, which causes biochemical changes in the cells. Choosing low-carbohydrate foods is one of the best ways to decrease inflammation. When blood sugar rises, sugar attaches to collagen in a process called glycosylation, which increases inflammation (and wrinkles!). Athletes mistakenly eat too many carbohydrates, which hinders their healing and recovery time because they are constantly inflaming their joints.

- **Sugar/glucose/fruit:** Sugar hinders the immune system, which also worsens fibromyalgia and chronic fatigue. The phagocytic index (a measurement of the number of bacteria ingested per phagocyte) tells you how rapidly a phagocyte (a cell that protects the body against foreign particles) can gobble up a virus, bacteria, or cancer cell. Because glucose and vitamin C have similar chemical structures, they compete with one another for entering cells when sugar levels go up. If more glucose is present, less vitamin C is allowed into the cell. It doesn't take much glucose to mediate the amount of vitamin C that enters your cells; a blood sugar value of 120 reduces the phagocytic index by 75 percent (meaning that the phagocytes' ability to remove foreign particles is reduced). When you eat sugar, your immune system slows to a crawl. Sugar is disguised as sucrose, corn syrup, and maltodextrin in our modern food supply. Fruits and fruit juices contain a lot of sugar. Sugar also increases blood sugar, which causes inflammation and pain.

- **Hormones and liver function:** The ways we get too much estrogen include being exposed to chemicals that mimic estrogen, such as those found in many plastics (microwaving food in plastic dishes or using plastic wraps and containers), and eating non-organic foods. Cows and chickens are typically given potent estrogenic substances (super-estrogens) to make them grow bigger faster. People develop estrogen dominance from eating a high-carb diet, consuming excess fructose, drinking alcohol, having a tired-toxic (chronically overloaded) liver, or being exposed to environmental toxins—all of which we have some power to control. The liver is a filter of sorts; it detoxifies our bodies, protecting us from the harmful effects of chemicals, elements in food, environmental toxins, and even natural products of our metabolism, including excess estrogen. Anything that impairs liver function or ties up the detoxifying function will result in excess estrogen levels. Detoxing the liver with ketogenic eating and castor oil packs and balancing your hormones with supplements will help the healing process.

- *Candida:* An overgrowth of yeast can cause muscle and joint pain, difficulty concentrating, chronic fatigue, neurological disorders, insomnia, bowel dysfunction, and a weakened immune system. These symptoms are similar to those of fibromyalgia. If you have been on antibiotics, have low moods, and crave carbs and sugar, you could have an overgrowth of yeast. A low-carb, low-sugar diet along with the correct probiotics can help kill the yeast. Eliminating foods that can cause *Candida* to grow—even mushrooms and moldy cheeses—is also necessary.

- **Excitotoxins:** Monosodium glutamate (MSG) and aspartame (NutraSweet or Equal) are excitotoxins to our brains, and everyone should eliminate them. Excitotoxins are found in just about every boxed and packaged food out there—even children's vitamins! They excite the neurons in the brain, causing them to fire so rapidly that they die. Once these cells are dead, they can't be remade. When you eliminate these food additives, symptoms initially get worse because your body detoxifies and releases the toxic substrates from their cells into the bloodstream.

- **Phosphates:** Most fibrous foods such as seeds, wheat, and oats contain phytic acid. Many people with chronic fatigue syndrome and fibromyalgia have a genetic defect that prevents their kidneys from excreting phosphates. The phosphates build up in the bones and eventually the muscles, ligaments, and tendons. The high level of phosphates damages the cells' ability to produce ATP (adenosine triphosphate, or cellular energy) and causes the muscles to spasm.

- **Free radicals:** An abundance of oxidative damage to the cells can cause fibromyalgia and chronic fatigue. When you are keto-adapted, there is less oxidative damage. A well-formulated ketogenic diet doesn't damage your immune system and creates less free radical damage in your cells. Free radicals are highly reactive molecules produced in the mitochondria that damage protein tissues and membranes of the cells. Free radicals develop as we exercise. However, ketones are a clean-burning fuel. When ketones are the fuel source, ROSs (oxygen free radicals) are drastically reduced. Intense exercise on a high-carb diet overwhelms the antioxidant defenses and cell membranes, which explains why extreme athletes often have impaired immune systems and decreased gut (intestinal) health. A well-formulated ketogenic diet fights off these aging antioxidants, reduces inflammation of the gut, and makes immune systems stronger than ever. Restoring the cells and eliminating free radicals is essential, and eating a well-formulated keto diet will accomplish this.

- **Food allergies:** Eliminate gluten, dairy, and soy. These common allergens cause an autoimmune response and often cause fibromyalgia and pain.

- **Nightshades:** Another possible source of pain comes from nightshade plants. Vegetables such as tomatoes, hot peppers, eggplant, and potatoes (not that we recommend potatoes for anyone) contain a chemical alkaloid called solanine, a type of poison. Solanine can trigger pain in some people. If you have persistent pain, we suggest eliminating these foods for one month to see what happens.

- **Other tips:** Get quality REM sleep, balance your omega-3 to omega-6 ratio by consuming healthy fish and quality egg yolks, boost your immune system, and get checked for parasites, which damage the immune system.

SUPPLEMENTS

Magnesium glycinate: Magnesium is a miracle mineral, and about 70 percent of people are deficient (mainly because it takes 54 milligrams of magnesium to process just 1 gram of sugar or starch!). Insulin stores magnesium, but if your insulin receptors are blunted and your cells grow resistant to insulin, you can't store magnesium, so it passes out of your body through urination. Magnesium in your cells relaxes your muscles. If your magnesium level is too low, your muscles constrict rather than relax, which increases pain and decreases energy. Supplement with 800 milligrams daily.

Vitamin D: Take 1,000 IU per 25 pounds of body weight if your vitamin D level is below 45. Read more about vitamin D in the "High Blood Pressure" section on pages 123 to 125.

Vitamin B12 and iron: Having a food allergy inhibits the intestines from absorbing iron and vitamin B12, both of which are essential for energy production. When we inhale, we carry oxygen through the hemoglobin to the mitochondria of our cells that burn fat and create energy. If we are deficient in iron, we can't carry the oxygen to the mitochondria. However, make sure you are low in iron before you begin taking supplements. Never take iron supplements unless you know you are low. Work with a healthcare professional to determine what dose to take and when to take it based on your current iron levels.

GLA (gamma-linolenic acid): GLA contains the pain-relieving compound phenylalanine and is increasingly being used to treat chronic pain. The nutrients in the GLA are essential for skin health, skin elasticity, and cellular structure. These fatty acids regulate hormones, including the thyroid and sex hormones. They also improve nerve function and cognition. Women should take 1,500 milligrams of emu oil or 1,300 milligrams of evening primrose oil three times a day with food. Men should take 600 milligrams of borage oil three times a day with food.

CANCER

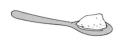

Why are the rates of cancer going up? In 1840, the average American consumed 2 tablespoons of sugar a day; by 2011, that number had grown to more than 63 tablespoons! Cancer loves glucose, which is why doctors test cancer patients by having them drink a "glucose" mix and then watch which cells consume that glucose the quickest (cancer is the fastest). You might think that you just need to cut glucose from your diet—and you are correct—but most people don't understand where all the glucose is coming from.

Glucose comes from more than just sugar. Structurally, complex carbohydrates are just glucose molecules joined together in long chains. The digestive tract breaks down those complex carbs into glucose. That means a sugary diet and a starchy diet are pretty much the same thing. In essence, a bowl of oatmeal, skim milk, and a banana is just a huge bowl of sugar. For about five years, German doctors have been testing cancer patients in a clinical study with a surprising prescription: fat. Their patients are on a ketogenic diet, which eliminates almost all carbohydrates and sugar and provides energy only from high-quality fats.

A well-formulated ketogenic diet has an intense and fast effect on cancer. All your body's cells can run on either glucose or FFA (free fatty acids). However, cancer cells have one huge flaw: They do not have the metabolic adaptability to be fueled by ketones; they can be fueled only by glucose. Because cancer cells need glucose to thrive and carbohydrates turn into glucose in the body, cutting out carbs can help starve the cancer cells.

On 02/15/13 I was diagnosed with a 12mm pineal gland cyst after a severe migraine. In late July, I flew to Colorado in hope of finding some answers and second opinions. Only more bad news followed. Not only was the cyst causing problems, but I was also on my way to getting type 2 diabetes and leaky gut. I knew I needed to change my life and fast. I found out about 'The Maria Way' from some very good friends. I have been sugar and gluten free since the beginning of August. [After] just 2.5 short weeks of being GF, I had my follow-up MRI. It showed that the cyst was now only 11mm in size. It had already shrunk by 1mm! I know that sounds tiny, but when you're talking about something growing in the middle of your brain, it means a lot! I have never felt better! Not only am I losing weight, but very soon I will be completely healthy! Thank you, Maria!

—Megan

You might be thinking that this advice runs contrary to the cancer diets you've heard about that focus on juicing and raw foods. However, scientific evidence supporting a carb-free diet as a means of fighting cancer dates back more than eighty years. In 1924, Nobel Prize winner Otto Warburg published his observations of a common feature he saw in fast-growing tumors. Unlike healthy cells that can get energy by metabolizing sugar in the mitochondria, cancer cells appeared to fuel themselves only through glycolysis, a less-efficient means of creating energy through the fermentation of sugar in the cytoplasm. This means they can run only on glucose. Warburg believed that this metabolic switch was the primary cause of cancer, a theory that he was unable to prove before he died in 1970.

If most aggressive cancers rely on the fermentation of sugar to grow and divide, then taking away the sugar can stop the cancer from spreading. Meanwhile, normal body and brain cells switch to generate energy from fatty molecules called ketones and FFA, the body's main source of energy on a fat-rich diet.

One theory that mistakenly sticks with cancer patients is that diet can influence pH balance. Tumor cells release lactic acid as a by-product, and this became known as the alkalinity-acidity theory. A number of books wrongly encourage alkaline diets for preventing and curing cancer. In reality, cancer cells are a bit more acidic just outside their boundaries than inside due to the expelling of lactic acid. Trying to control the pH in your body appears to be unhelpful. The absence of acid in the gastric tract and bladder establishes an environment that is favorable to tumor growth. Also, the control of pH is automatically kept in a tight range that is a neutral 7.2 to 7.4. Our diets have been proven to have little to no effect on blood pH.

A ketogenic diet is helpful for cancer patients for many reasons:

- It decreases the buildup of lactate, which helps control pH and respiratory function. A myth about low-carb diets is that they put you in a state of ketoacidosis. This misconception stems from the fact that many doctors confuse nutritional ketosis with diabetic ketoacidosis (DKA). Nutritional ketosis is marked by a blood ketone range of 0.5 to about 5.0 mmol, with low blood sugar levels. DKA is 15 mmol or higher, with very high blood glucose, which results in an acidic environment in the body. This state really only occurs when type 1 diabetics are not managing their insulin properly, and it's a very different state from nutritional ketosis.

- A ketogenic diet doesn't damage the immune system, and it creates less free radical damage in our cells compared to a high-carb diet. Free radicals are highly reactive molecules produced in the mitochondria that damage protein tissues and membranes of the cells. Free radicals develop as we exercise. But ketones and FFA are clean-burning fuel. When ketones and FFA are the fuel source, ROS (reactive oxygen species) are drastically reduced. Intense exercise on a high-carb diet overwhelms the antioxidant defenses and cell membranes, which explains why some extreme athletes have impaired immune systems and decreased gut health. A well-designed ketogenic diet fights off these aging free radicals and reduces inflammation in the gut, making immune systems stronger than ever.

- Researchers are increasingly looking at cancer as a metabolic disease, and a ketogenic diet is seen as a way to convert the body to an environment that inhibits cancer instead of promoting its growth (like a high-sugar diet does).

Two common imbalances—in the minerals zinc and selenium—are known to increase the rate of cancer.

ZINC IMBALANCE

Let us grab your attention by telling you that zinc is required for collagen development and protein synthesis. Zinc deficiency is often the cause of sagging skin that has lost its elasticity. If you have thin, peeling, and brittle nails or white spots on your nails, you are likely deficient in zinc. You lose a lot of zinc as you sweat. Zinc deficiency is also related to cancer because it is needed for a healthy immune system.

Lactating women need large amounts of zinc. If a nursing mother is lacking in zinc, the consequence can be impaired development and growth of the infant. When a woman is deficient in zinc or zinc isn't accurately metabolized, breast cancer is often a result. Low levels of zinc activate breast cancer cells and can cause the cancer to spread at an alarming rate. Zinc deficiencies cause compromised cellular functioning in the breast because there is a cluster of proteins gathered around a zinc ion that binds to a woman's DNA and affects gene regulation.

Low zinc leads to excess copper levels, which make the breasts more sensitive to the effects of excessive bad estrogen. Zinc supports the production and use of progesterone. Without adequate progesterone to balance out excess estrogen, estrogen dominance starts to develop, which causes an increased risk of estrogen-dominant cancers, such as breast, ovarian, uterine, thyroid, and prostate cancers.

Ketogenic foods that are high in zinc include egg yolks, lamb, liver, beef, poultry, sardines, oysters, and other seafood.

SELENIUM IMBALANCE

Getting adequate selenium is also helpful in combating the formation of cancer because of the effect selenium has on the genes involved in cellular processes. Selenium's greatest effect is its power over the genes that order circadian rhythm. It also lowers the oxidation of fats and boosts the immune system.

Selenium is essential for the conversion of T4 to T3, the active form of thyroid hormone that helps lower autoimmune responses, especially after giving birth. During pregnancy, the immune system goes into overdrive to protect the fetus. After the baby is born, women often develop antibodies against the thyroid. Adding 200 micrograms of selenium daily helps lower this immune response.

Selenium is found in beef, liver, chicken, salmon, and seafood. Brazil nuts contain the highest amounts. In fact, two Brazil nuts contain about 200 micrograms. However, to ensure you get an adequate amount of selenium, we suggest supplementing daily.

MODIFICATIONS

Eat only high-quality organic and pastured sources of animal protein.

Consider fasting to purge unhealthy cells. Fast well, feast well, as we like to say. Many studies have shown that fasting can be very effective at stopping cancer growth and even reversing it through increased apoptosis (programmed cell death). See Chapter 9 for more on fasting.

Cut out all sugar and carbs, because sugar depresses the immune system. White blood cells need vitamin C so that they can phagocytize viruses and bacteria. White blood cells require a fifty times higher concentration of vitamin C inside the cell as outside, which means they must accumulate the vitamin. The phagocytic index tells you how rapidly a lymphocyte can gobble up a virus, bacteria, or cancer cell. It doesn't take much; a blood sugar value of 120 reduces the phagocytic index by 75 percent. When you eat whole grains and sugar, your immune system slows to a crawl. Because sugar lacks minerals and vitamins, they draw upon the body's micronutrient stores to be metabolized by the system.

Consider hyperbaric oxygen treatment. Some studies have shown that a ketogenic diet in addition to hyperbaric oxygen treatment can help treat some cancers.[14]

SUPPLEMENTS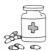

Bifidobacteria: Seventy percent of the immune system comes from the gut. Keep it healthy with probiotics. Take one capsule of *Bifidobacteria* daily with a tablespoon of coconut vinegar or a can of sardines for prebiotics.

Glutathione: Glutathione is a super-antioxidant for cellular health. Take 500 milligrams at each meal.

CoQ10: CoQ10 builds mitochondria. Supplement with 400 milligrams with your first meal of the day.

Alpha-lipoic acid (ALA): Alpha-lipoic acid is a neuroprotective antioxidant that can cross the blood-brain barrier. Take 400 milligrams once daily with food. (Make sure to choose a German source; Chinese sources often contain harmful additives.)

Zinc: Zinc is essential for creating DNA, supporting the immune system, building proteins, and triggering enzymes. It also helps cells communicate by functioning as a neurotransmitter. Zinc can cause nausea, so start with 10 milligrams once per day, with your first meal of the day, for one week. Increase by 10 milligrams each week until you can take 50 milligrams without feeling nauseated.

Vitamin D: Vitamin D helps build bones. Take 1,000 IU per 25 pounds of body weight if your level is below 45. Read more about vitamin D in the "High Blood Pressure" section (pages 123 to 125).

EstroFactors: EstroFactors is especially good for treating prostate, thyroid, breast, and uterine cancers. EstroFactors is a unique formula designed to detox excess bad estrogen; it works for men and boys, too. Take three capsules.

Gamma-linoleic acid (GLA): GLA helps lower estrogen dominance. GLA is essential for skin health, skin elasticity, and cellular structure. These fatty acids regulate hormones, including thyroid and sex hormones. They also improve nerve function and cognition. Women should take 1,500 milligrams of emu oil or 1,300 milligrams of evening primrose oil three times a day with food. Men should take 600 milligrams of borage oil three times a day with food.

Selenium: Getting adequate selenium is a helpful step in combating the formation of cancer because of its effect on the levels of genes involved in cellular processes. Supplement with 200 micrograms daily, with or without food.

Our family discovered the 'Maria Way' a few years ago, but we had not fully put it into practice. A little over a year ago, tragedy hit when we discovered our three-year-old boy had a five-pound cancerous tumor attached to his kidney. After major surgery and a five-day hospital stay, we knew we needed to change our nutrition. If there were ever a time for taking drastic measure, it was then. We consulted with Maria and cleaned out every ounce of sugar and grains from our house.

Our young family of four all adopted a new way of eating, a new way of life. Since I have such a loving, committed wife who took care of most of the cooking, you could say I was more or less along for the ride. I was surprised to find that this journey had many unexpected benefits right from the start.

When we began eating the 'Maria Way,' I weighed in at over 200 pounds. Just a few months later I had lost just over 40 pounds. I have had multiple knee surgeries and suffer from arthritis and joint pain. However since we kicked the grains and sugar, I have little to no soreness ever. Stairs were an issue and no longer are. I sleep through the night regularly now, and my energy level is through the roof. You could say the kids also had this same benefit!

Though this way of eating (menu planning/prep work/etc.) can be difficult at times, it has brought our family together in love, and in the kitchen! Our son has been doing fantastic with perfect check-ups. Our family has been learning about new foods and how to be better cooks, and we could not have done it without Maria's help.

—Joe

Ketone supplements: Ketone supplements may be beneficial for dealing with cancer. Much research is ongoing, led by Dr. Dominic D'Agostino at the University of Southern Florida.

METABOLIC SYNDROME AND TYPE 2 DIABETES

"

My father-in-law has type 2 diabetes and is not fond of trying new foods. Maybe [it's] due to being picky but [it's] also because he has had terrible diabetes for over thirty years. My father-in-law has large blood sugar swings even with his insulin pump.

He tried [Maria's] waffles and muffins and loved them. Keep in mind he had butter on both and sugar-free syrup on the waffle. As we stood in the kitchen discussing how many units of insulin he should calculate for the food he ate, we came to the conclusion that he should take five units. Normally for the food he had just consumed he would have needed to take eight, but since Maria's food is different we shot it on the lower side. . . . My father-in-law left for about one hour and came back out of sorts. My mother-in-law said, 'Tom, are you OK . . . go check your blood.' He checked his blood and it had taken a huge nosedive . . . he had a blood sugar level of 45! Now at this time only two units had gone into his body . . . not five, and he had to stop the rest of the insulin from entering his system. We couldn't believe it! Here he had taken almost four times less than he normally would have and his levels were too low.

Now he doesn't need any insulin to maintain his blood sugar levels!

—Cindy

Type 2 diabetes and metabolic disease are becoming epidemics in America. As discussed in Chapter 2, the root cause of insulin resistance is the overstuffed and inflamed adipose tissue (fat cells). To reverse insulin resistance, we must get into a negative fat flux (burn more fat than is being stored) as quickly as we can. Burning more fat and shrinking the fat cells restores insulin signaling and can enable you to have A1c levels and fasting glucose that are no longer in the diabetic range.

My grandpa was a type 2 diabetic, and I was so frustrated with the way they fed him at his assisted living facility. Who came up with these plans and guidelines? Mine is just a little voice compared to the large diabetic association, but stories like my grandfather's remind me of the fable "The Starfish":

A young man was walking along the shore after a storm. Many starfish had washed up on the beach during the storm, and the young man was taking the time to return them to the sea. An older man observed this and said, "But, young man, don't you realize that there are miles and miles of beach and starfish all along it? You can't possibly make a difference!"

The young man listened politely. Then he bent down, picked up another starfish, and threw it into the sea, past the breaking waves, and said, "It made a difference for that one."

MODIFICATIONS

Eat a well-formulated ketogenic diet and spread protein out over your meals. Depending on how much insulin resistance you have, you might want to consider spreading out your protein over your meals. You still want to hit your protein goal; just don't get too much protein in one meal.

Add cold thermogenesis (cold therapy). This increases the amount of brown fat. The more brown fat you have, the more glucose it uses lowering blood glucose levels.

Add intermittent fasting and try protein-sparing modified fasting (PSMF). This can help shrink fat cells faster and restore insulin signaling faster.

SUPPLEMENTS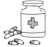

Berberine: Berberine has been shown to help reduce blood sugar levels in some diabetics. Supplement with 1,000 milligrams twice a day.

Vitamin D. Optimize your vitamin D levels, which helps boost the immune system. Read more about vitamin D in the "High Blood Pressure" section (pages 123 to 125).

Magnesium glycinate: Magnesium is a miracle mineral, and about 70 percent of people are deficient in their magnesium levels (mainly because it takes 54 milligrams of magnesium to process 1 gram of sugar/starch!). Insulin stores magnesium, but if your insulin receptors are blunted and your cells grow resistant to insulin, you can't store magnesium, so it passes out of your body through urination. Magnesium in your cells relaxes muscles. If your magnesium level is too low, your muscles will constrict rather than relax, which increases pain and decreases your energy level. Take 800 milligrams daily.

Zinc: Zinc is essential for creating DNA, supporting a healthy immune system, building proteins, and triggering enzymes. It also helps cells communicate by functioning as a neurotransmitter. As previously noted, taking zinc can make you nauseated, so we recommend starting slowly and ramping up your dosage by 10 milligrams a week until you can take 50 milligrams once a day without being nauseated. Take zinc with your first meal of the day.

TYPE 1 DIABETES

We work with a lovely woman with type 1 diabetes who said, "I wish I would gain weight when I cheat. We are a vain society. I know that I have internal inflammation, but since I don't see it on the outside, I have a hard time staying on your keto meal plans."

She was right. She had terrible internal inflammation. Her A1c was 11.5, and she'd had a stroke. Jennifer was only twenty-eight and had just had a baby girl for whom she needed to stay healthy, but her addiction to carbs and sugar was getting the best of her. She also was right when she said we are a vain society. It isn't until we look unhealthy on the outside that we finally change our poor eating habits.

Type 1 diabetes affects many people, and most doctors do little to help control it other than to add more and more insulin without changing the patient's diet. However, it is very important to use diet to reduce insulin needs. Reducing insulin improves health in the long run and leads to lower A1c and blood sugar levels.

We get comments and letters from a lot of type 1 diabetics who say that we need to remember to refer to type 2 diabetes when we write about carbohydrates and our clients' success stories. We understand the differences between type 1 and type 2 diabetes, but a well-formulated ketogenic diet helps type 1 diabetes, too! Type 1 diabetes develops when antibodies destroy the cells in the pancreas that produce and secrete insulin. The body normally produces these antibodies to defend itself from foreign invaders, but sometimes these helpful antibodies turn on the body's cells. In the case of type 1 diabetes, the antibodies target the pancreatic cells. Most of the time, these antibodies can be identified through the examination of a blood sample. When antibodies are present in the blood, it means the blood is attacking a foreign substance. When food leaks from the intestines into the bloodstream (because of leaky gut), the blood reacts by attacking the protein found in foods, such as the gluten found in wheat or the casein found in dairy. In this case, we need to lower the autoimmune response as well as count carbohydrates. This is why a high-fat, adequate-protein, low-carb, and allergen-free diet works for autoimmune disorders. It eliminates the proteins that cause the autoimmune response and lowers the carbs so the body can heal. There have been several studies showing an association between type 1 diabetes and celiac disease, and we have seen awesome results when eliminating gluten and carbs.

If you have type 1 diabetes and you start eating a well-formulated ketogenic diet, it is extremely important to work closely with your doctor. Some clients tell us that their doctors say things like, "Don't worry. Eat whatever you want. Just make sure you cover your glucose with insulin." We think this is like saying to a firefighter, "Don't worry. Pour as much gasoline as you like on that fire, as long as you cover it with enough water." This way of thinking is dangerous and irrational. If your doctor has a similar theory, we suggest finding a new doctor who will encourage you to eat a ketogenic diet while watching your need for insulin.

We have helped many people with type 1 diabetes realize A1c levels below 5.0! Following the keto lifestyle and adjusting your insulin as needed can result in very good blood sugar control.

MODIFICATIONS

Eat a well-formulated ketogenic diet and spread out protein over your meals. You still want to hit your protein goal; just don't get too much protein at any one meal. You also want to get enough insulin to cover the protein to ensure that it is properly utilized. Typically, that is about one-half the bolus amount you use for carbohydrates, which ensures there is enough insulin for your body to use the protein.

> **TIP**
>
> A Facebook group called Typeonegrit focuses on people who manage their type 1 diabetes with diet. This group is a great resource for learning how to adjust your insulin and adapt to a keto lifestyle.

Add cold thermogenesis (cold therapy). Cold therogenesis increases brown fat. The more brown fat you have, the more glucose it uses, lowering your blood glucose levels.

SUPPLEMENTS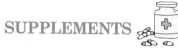

Berberine: In some diabetics, berberine has been shown to help reduce blood sugar levels. Take 1,000 milligrams twice a day.

> *I'd like to preface this with a little background info. I am a type 1 diabetic who has been following an essentially ketogenic diet since 2012. Since that time, my blood sugars have improved dramatically by following the dietary recommendations of Richard K. Bernstein (another devout low-carb advocate). But while carrying a consistent A1c of 4.8–5.0 these past years is a spectacular blessing, and I follow the diet religiously, I find the diet itself rather limiting.*
>
> *This is where your work has come into play in my life. I'd recently discovered your* Art of Eating Healthy *books on Kindle and was so impressed, I downloaded* Sweets *and bought one more. Your work has gone such a long way toward offering a sense of normalcy to my diet. Food used to be my way to reach out to the world. I would cook when stressed, and it added such a sense of success to my life. When I switched to extreme low carb in 2012, I lost much of that outlet in my life. But now, I am enjoying ketogenic breads, wonderful high fat, low-carb dessert options as well as an array of things to re-experience. (Brown gravy over mashed cauliflower, yes, please!)*
>
> *I've always been lean, but I now carry more muscle than I've ever been able to. And while I imagine that most people must thank you for health-related outcomes, I am going to offer thanks for restoring a sense of normalcy and enthusiasm for a part of my life I missed . . . not to mention attaining marked pleasure and satisfaction from my meals.*
>
> *From the bottom of my heart, thank you for your work in the ketogenic world—it improves the quality and enjoyment of my life. Even if there was some miraculous cure to diabetes, I would still eat this way for the rest of my life if that tells you anything. You've done so much to influence my cooking in such a short time.*

—Chris

chapter 7

Common Mistakes

There is a lot of confusion about what constitutes a well-formulated ketogenic diet. When it comes to keto, there are three main camps:

- One camp thinks that as long as a person's macros (percentages of carbs, fat, and protein) are good, the source of the food doesn't matter. This group believes that it's okay to get those macros from fast food, processed foods, and the like. We call this the "junk food keto" group.
- Another camp thinks that you need to eat much more fat and limit protein.
- The third camp thinks that you need to keep carbs low and get enough protein for your lean mass and use fat as a lever to lose, maintain, or gain weight, depending on your goal.

Obviously, we are in the third camp, but let's take a look at the other two and make it clear why we believe proponents of those ideologies are mistaken and why those approaches can be harmful or hold you back from the results you are seeking.

The "junk food keto" group is just trading one problem for another. All the chemicals, preservatives, food dyes, omega-6 seed and vegetable oils, and other junk contained in processed foods cause problems and inflammation. People in this camp might lose weight, but ingesting these junk foods affects their healing and longevity, and it puts an extra load on liver detoxing. We believe that a whole-foods approach enables much more healing and weight loss by reducing the burden on our livers.

For the keto "experts" who think that consuming more fat and less protein is the way to go, we created a list of common myths, which are covered in the following sections.

When I write about my past mistakes, including eating carbs on the weekends, I am not judging anyone for having 'cheat days.' My words come from a place of love and are meant to encourage you. I certainly do not want to give you permission to cheat. To me, giving a carb addict permission to eat carbs on cheat days is no different than telling an alcoholic that it's okay to have just one drink. I want you to know that listening to those bad messages of 'I was craving it, so my body must need it' held me back for years, and it will hold you back, too. Allowing myself to have more carbs on the weekends held me back from healing my polycystic ovary syndrome (PCOS). By adding carbs on the weekends, you keep going into that awful state of 'carb withdrawal,' which is often mistakenly called the 'keto flu.'

My sugar addiction started at a young age, and it was a hard addiction to break. It was even harder for Craig. I had to sit through many date night dinners with French fries and decadent desserts staring me in the face. I never nagged him. Instead, I just led by example, and I'm grateful that he eventually changed. We grew together instead of apart. I often hear clients say, 'My husband will never do this lifestyle with me.' But I say, 'Never say never!' Before going keto, Craig brewed his own beer and made his own wine. He doesn't drink either of them anymore. He is a completely different man than the man I fell in love with at age seventeen, but I love him even more now.

You need to start thinking positive. Instead of thinking the glass is half-empty, you need to start thinking that the glass is half full! You can't think about all the foods you can't have. Think about all the amazing foods you can have! You have the power to change your palate. I was the pickiest eater! I made my best friend Marla's mother cry at dinner because I never ate her food. I have overcome my love for junk, and you can, too!

If you truly want to heal, get off medication, and stop feeling ill, you need to stop adding carbs, which will just set you back. We had a client contact us after a year of no contact, and she admitted she innocently started adding sweet potatoes, which led to carb cravings and eating more and more carbs, and that led to a 30-pound weight gain.

You know how you often overeat at a buffet or a potluck? I do, too! Having too much variety in flavors stimulates overeating. Your mind gets bored by a certain flavor, so you then move on to the next tasty flavor on your plate. Limiting different flavors helps control eating behavior. I recently spoke at a clinic in New York, and the doctor told his patients to stop eating so much variety! He eats a rib-eye and some keto ice cream every night (there are many keto ice cream recipes in my cookbooks and on my website, mariamindbodyhealth.com).

When you have setbacks, please know that we never judge you. Food can be an addiction. We believe it is one of the hardest addictions to overcome because eating is unavoidable. You need to eat.

Let food be thy medicine.

—Maria

DISPELLING KETO MYTHS

In this section, we dispel some common myths about the keto lifestyle.

MYTH 1: KETO IS ALL ABOUT HORMONES; CALORIES DON'T MATTER

This one we must unpack a bit because it is somewhat complicated. First, calories do matter. However, we are not saying we are back to the old calories-in, calories-out way of thinking. Hormones matter, too. They both matter! And restoring proper hormone signaling is one of the great aspects of a well-formulated ketogenic diet. When you restore proper hormone signaling, you reduce hunger and cravings, which makes eating less much easier (enabling more fat loss).

As described in Chapters 2 and 3, insulin signaling breakdown occurs when too many of your fat cells get overstuffed and inflamed. To reverse this, you must reduce the size of these fat cells by enabling lipolysis (pulling fat from fat stores to be used as fuel). Fuel—even fat—coming in through the foods you eat raises insulin levels enough to shut off lipolysis and stop the shrinking of the fat cells that is so important for healing. In fact, when you consume excess fat, your fat cells are enlarged.

When you are keto-adapted, you can use your dietary fat and body fat equally. You want your body to use stored body fat for fuel so that you lose excess body fat.

That means while we are not saying this is the same old calories in, calories out way of thinking, we are also not saying that calories don't matter. Hormones are important, but so are calories. They both matter!

MYTH 2: SLEEP, HORMONE, OR THYROID ISSUES REQUIRE ADDITIONAL CARBS

Carb-ups involve adding carbs in the evening, supposedly to help with various issues. Some people believe that doing carb-ups helps with sleep, hormones, and thyroid function, among other things. However, carb-ups just cover up the real issues, and it's plain wrong to think that carb-ups are necessary.

Hormone signaling isn't restored overnight. It takes time. The keto lifestyle will help get your body back into a natural hormone balance—you just need to give it time. Adding carbs just sets you back, introduces cravings, or, even worse, starts a carb binge. You are much better off to address the root cause and take some supplements to help balance out your hormones more quickly while sticking to a ketogenic diet. For more information about how to make modifications for different conditions, see Chapter 6.

Also, carb-ups or carb-cycling on the weekends leads to more lean mass loss, and you definitely don't want that. A deep keto state is where you start preserving your lean mass. With carb-ups, you end up in a kind of in-between state in which your body isn't fully keto-adapted but also isn't getting enough carbohydrates to be a full sugar burner. Consequently, you use more lean protein to satisfy the glucose needs, which leads to loss of lean mass.

People who advocate this carb-up approach say things like, "I eat 80 grams of carbs but stay in ketosis." This is related to myth 5, "High Blood Ketones Equal Nutritional Ketosis." These same people advocate lots of fat bombs, bulletproof coffee, and lots of other added fat. As we describe in myth 5, this isn't nutritional ketosis. You have elevated ketones because of the large amounts of external fat, not because you're making them from your fat stores (which is what you want for true nutritional ketosis and fat loss). Also, it doesn't mean much when you test for ketones in the morning after having had a carb-up the night before. After twelve hours of not eating (overnight), most people show some elevated ketones, whether they are ketosis or not.

As Dr. Steven Phinney, one of the most respected researchers on ketogenic lifestyles, says, "Forcing the pancreas to make more insulin by eating more carbs clearly doesn't do a lot of good for type 2 diabetics, and we think the same logic applies here for thyroid function."[1]

Keto is very low-carb for a reason. Adding carbs would just mess up all the healing that keto can provide. Stop chasing ketones and chase results.

MYTH 3: NOT ALL FAT IS ABSORBED WHEN YOU'RE KETO

This one is pretty abstract and isn't supported by any biology or evolutionary facts. The idea is that not all the fat you eat gets absorbed; when you're in ketosis, lots of it just goes through you and into the stool. There are three important points about this myth:

- Studies have shown that only about 5 grams of fat a day is passed through the stool.[2] The rest is either stored or used as fuel.

- Do you remember Olestra? It was a fake, processed oil produced in the 1990s and used in potato chips. The big "benefit" was that the oil didn't get digested, which meant that you really did just poop it out. The makers of Olestra had to include a warning label stating that it could cause abdominal cramping, loose stools, and even uncontrolled anal leakage! And those side effects would come from maybe 5 to 10 grams of extra fat going out the digestive tract. We can't imagine what would happen if you truly had 100 grams of fat just "going out" because being keto means you don't absorb the fat. We don't think we would want that uncontrollable result.

- This last point comes from an evolutionary perspective. If we didn't absorb the fats we ate, we wouldn't be around as a species. Hunter-gathers ate lots of animal fats in the summer months to add extra body fat to make it through the lean winters. If we didn't use all this wonderful energy coming into our bodies, that wouldn't be a very smart biological system. Life doesn't just waste energy. If anything, it holds onto every bit it can so you can make it through the lean times.

MYTH 4: EATING FAT DURING A FAST WON'T BREAK YOUR FAST

Fat is calories. The whole point of fasting and intermittent fasting is not to have any calories to enable your body to do repair activities (autophagy and apoptosis; see Chapter 9 for details) and utilize more stored body fat for fuel. If you add calories you raise insulin, which means the process stops and so do the benefits. Any calories, including those from fat, raise insulin enough to stop lipolysis and decrease the benefits of fasting.

We believe the thinking behind this myth comes from the thought, "If I am showing high ketones, then my fast is okay." Again, having higher ketones does not mean better results. And for best results, fasting means no calories (water only).

MYTH 5: HIGH BLOOD KETONES EQUAL NUTRITIONAL KETOSIS

Nutritional ketosis means your body is making ketones to fuel your body and you are primarily running on stored body fat (free fatty acids and ketones). This only happens when carbs get low enough, and you spend less time stimulating insulin.

There are several things that can elevate blood ketones without it coming from your body (what you really want). These include coconut oil, MCT oil, MCT powders, and exogenous ketones. These all can raise blood ketones. You can eat a big bowl of rice loaded with MCT oil and still show "keto" blood ketone levels of, say, 0.5 mmol. However, you are not in nutritional ketosis. This myth is what leads some to say, "I eat 80 grams of carbs a day and am in ketosis." They are just adding lots and lots of fats to keep blood ketones elevated a bit. They are not in nutritional ketosis, and they aren't using body fat for fuel. Don't chase ketones; chase results!

MYTH 6: HIGHER KETONES ARE BETTER

There is no correlation between blood ketone levels and weight loss and healing. High ketones don't mean greater weight loss. There are some cases where higher blood ketones are beneficial, such as with Alzheimer's disease or for dealing with seizures. But if weight loss and healing are your goal, then more is not necessarily better.

Blood ketones are simply the difference in fuel generated and fuel used. If you are active and have been in ketosis for a while, you can have low ketones even if you're eating few to zero carbs. That is because your body is using the ketones for fuel, which is leaving fewer ketones in the bloodstream. We know bodybuilders who are very keto and never have blood ketones much above 0.3 mmol or so. Focus on getting carbs low enough, and you will be in ketosis regardless of what your fat intake is, and regardless of what your blood ketones say. Remember: Don't chase ketones; chase results!

MYTH 7: EXOGENOUS KETONES WILL HELP WITH WEIGHT LOSS

As shown in Chapter 3, any fuel coming into the body stops lipolysis, which makes perfect sense. If your body wants to tightly control the amount of fuel in the blood at any given time, it must stop adding fuel to the blood as soon as any comes in through the diet. This is the same argument as the next myth about adding fat when weight loss stalls. You want your body to be making ketones from your body fat rather than making ketones from dietary fat for fuel. You know what we're going to say, right? Don't chase ketones; chase results!

MYTH 8: IF YOU ARE STALLED, ADD MORE FAT

This advice is also common and is very flawed. There are some keto "experts" who give this damaging advice all too often. Not losing weight? Eat more fat. Losing hair? Eat more fat. Some people recommend lowering protein to dangerously low levels while raising fat. They tell people to get less than 50 grams of protein while eating 200 grams or more of fat! Chapter 8 makes clear why this is such bad advice. You are exchanging the most nutrient-dense food (animal protein) for one of the least nutrient-dense foods (fat). You are also using more and more dietary fat for fuel and using less and less body fat for fuel. This is the opposite of what you want for fat loss.

> " *If your body is already high fat, then all you need is low carb.*
>
> —Dr. Ted Naiman

MYTH 9: TOO MUCH PROTEIN TURNS INTO SUGAR

This is a widely held belief in the keto community, but it's another myth that doesn't have scientific or biological backing. Yes, there is a metabolic pathway for converting protein to glucose. It is called gluconeogenesis. However, that pathway is always on, meaning that when the body needs more glucose, it produces more glucose. Studies have shown that increases in protein intake have little or no effect on the rate of gluconeogenesis. In fact, most of the gluconeogenesis that occurs when you are keto-adapted is from glycerol. Remember our discussion of lipolysis in Chapter 3? The first step in lipolysis is where a triglyceride molecule has the glycerol stripped off, which frees three FFA molecules to enter the bloodstream to be used as fuel. The glycerol molecule is then sent to the liver; three glycerol molecules combine to form one glucose molecule.

Gluconeogenesis is not an enemy of a ketogenic diet; instead, gluconeogenesis is what makes a keto diet possible. With a carbohydrate intake of 20 grams or less per day, your body wouldn't have enough glucose to fuel the parts of your brain that can run only on glucose.

Gluconeogenesis makes the extra glucose needed to fuel the brain and thus makes a ketogenic diet possible.

Some people point out that type 1 diabetics must dose insulin at about one-half the rate of carbohydrates to prevent large blood glucose spikes. However, this isn't the result of gluconeogenesis. When you eat protein, both insulin and glucagon are released. Insulin is released to stimulate protein synthesis or the uptake of amino acids in muscle cells. This process makes them less available for gluconeogenesis. The glucagon is released to stimulate the uptake of amino acids into the liver for gluconeogenesis. The release of two competing hormones serves a very important purpose. A rise in insulin lowers blood sugar levels. A rise in glucagon raises blood sugar levels. In a non-diabetic, this ensures that the amino acids get used for protein synthesis but also ensures that blood sugar doesn't drop to dangerously low levels. That means the insulin and glucagon cancel each other out with respect to glucose levels while the insulin still acts on the protein to perform muscle synthesis. This is a pretty neat trick.

TYPEONEGRIT

Our friend R. D. Dikeman is an advocate for using a ketogenic lifestyle to help manage type 1 diabetes. He founded the group Typeonegrit that helps people manage their type 1 diabetes with diet and lifestyle. He often says, "Avoiding protein because of gluconeogenesis is like avoiding air because of asthma."

In a type 1 diabetic, the release of glucagon without insulin—type 1 diabetics don't produce insulin as they should—can cause a blood sugar rise after meals that are high in protein. Also, the absence of insulin increases the amount of protein used for gluconeogenesis because there isn't enough insulin to counter the rise of glucagon, which is why a diabetic needs to account for protein in insulin dosing.

Gluconeogenesis is what makes a ketogenic diet possible. It is always running and regulating our blood sugar levels, and it's mostly demand driven. If blood glucose goes low, the body makes more. It does have some supply variations (very high protein levels can produce excess protein that gets turned into more blood glucose), but the effect is minimal. Many people can eat 150 grams of protein in one sitting with a negligible effect on blood sugar. So protein is not the enemy of a ketogenic diet. And, as explained in Chapter 8, it can be the key to improving nutrient density in your diet.

MYTH 10: KETO REQUIRES 80 PERCENT FAT, 15 PERCENT PROTEIN, AND 5 PERCENT CARBS

The problem with this belief is that it is very dependent on calories. One person could be eating 3,000 calories, in which case the necessary protein would be 112 grams a day. A person eating 1,000 calories would need only 37 grams of protein a day to reach that 15 percent goal. We know that protein is dependent on lean mass: The more lean mass you have, the more protein you need to maintain it. That means you should always track your macros (fat, protein, and carbs) in grams, not percentages.

A well-formulated ketogenic diet is a whole-food, organic approach to keto with low carbs and adequate protein. Some people in the keto community are giving advice that is holding people back and even causing more damage. We hope we have cleared up some of the confusion about various myths.

If handled correctly, a well-formulated ketogenic diet can produce amazing results for weight loss and a wide range of chronic diseases. We have seen it firsthand in thousands of clients and with everything from Alzheimer's disease, multiple sclerosis, metabolic disease, cancer, autoimmune issues, thyroid problems,

KETO DIETS ARE LOW-CARB, HIGH-FAT DIETS

Ketogenic diets are often called low-carb, high-fat (LCHF) diets. The misinterpretation of this label is that the high fat must come from the diet. If you are overweight, you are already high fat. Let your body use the stored body fat instead supplying it with dietary fat.

and so much more. We believe that it's important to have clarity regarding what a well-formulated ketogenic diet really is because the stakes—your health—are really high.

If you are doing the things we outline for a well-formulated ketogenic diet and are still having trouble reaching your goals, the next section about troubleshooting might help you get the weight loss and healing going again.

TROUBLESHOOTING: WHY IT MIGHT NOT BE WORKING

We want to start out by reminding you that a well-formulated ketogenic diet is very specific with proper ratios, specific foods, extra electrolytes, and water. We often get clients who claim they eat keto but come to find that certain foods they are consuming are limiting their results and keeping them from the weight loss they desire.

A well-formulated ketogenic diet will not create the ill effects people experience when first going low-carb, such as feeling tired, feeling depressed, and having heavy legs when walking up stairs. These are the symptoms of the so-called "low-carb flu." A common mistake people make when they experience these symptoms is to start adding fruits, higher-carb veggies (such as spaghetti squash), and other carbohydrates to their diet because they "feel better" when they add carbs. However, the issue was that they didn't formulate the diet properly to begin with, and adding carbs just keeps them from fully keto-adapting. The real problem was that they were low in sodium and electrolytes, and adding carbs just made them retain water and electrolytes. When you first start a low-carb or ketogenic diet, you lose a lot of water weight (and electrolytes), and you need to supplement accordingly. See Chapter 4 for electrolyte recommendations.

When clients are adapting to the keto lifestyle, one of the first effects is a rapid improvement in insulin sensitivity. Eating low-carb causes insulin levels to fall quickly. As we mentioned earlier, as insulin levels fall, the kidneys begin to release fluid promptly. A common complaint we hear from clients when they first adopt this lifestyle is that they are up in the middle of the night urinating more than usual. This effect will go away with time, which is a good thing, but there is some bad news that comes along with it.

The good news is that when you release excess fluid, fat oxidation becomes easier. The bad news is that as the extra water goes, it also removes essential sodium and electrolytes. When sodium levels fall below a certain level, which can happen quite quickly, there are some undesirable side effects, such as headaches, low energy, dizziness, and cramping. Reread Chapter 4 to get the guidelines for a well-formulated ketogenic diet. If you follow those recommendations, you won't suffer from the low-carb flu, and your weight loss should get back on track.

COMMON KETO MISTAKES

We hope you don't run into any stalls and just keep losing weight and feeling better than ever. However, some people have more damaged metabolisms. The advice in this section can help you break through those stalls, overcome common pitfalls that limit results, and get things moving in the right direction again.

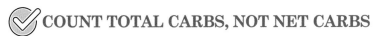 ## COUNT TOTAL CARBS, NOT NET CARBS

A common mistake is counting net carbs rather than total carbohydrates. Net carbs are total carbs minus fiber. Also, don't subtract fiber from vegetable carbohydrates. Our meal plans contain only the most nutrient-rich proteins and veggies without high total carb counts. We have many clients whose weight loss stalls when they consume too much fiber. This is common when people first try a ketogenic diet and eat too many nuts, nut flours, seeds, and psyllium. There are also ingredients listed as fiber that will spike blood sugar, such as inulin in protein bars. Counting total carbs is much safer, and it also makes tracking easier.

AVOID NUTS, NUT FLOURS, SEEDS, AND PSYLLIUM FOR WEIGHT LOSS

The ketogenic diet isn't just for weight loss. We have many clients who are trying to gain weight, put on muscle, or simply maintain good health. That is why we include recipes made with nut flours in our cookbooks and on our blog. However, our meal plans for weight loss are very specific and cut out all nuts, nut flours, seeds, and psyllium.

WHAT THE FLAX?

Many people make the mistake of adding lots of flax when going keto, but that's not a good idea, and the false and ignorant articles claiming flaxseeds are a superfood that heals all ailments remind us of the bad information we were sold when soy first entered the mass market.

First off, our traditional diet never included flax. Flax was used to make rope and linen. Later, the flax seeds were opened to make oil, but not the kind of oil you might be thinking of. The oil was used in paints and varnishes! Also, flax oil isn't saturated, so it goes rancid quickly.

Adding flax to your diet not only ups your carb intake but also adds a lot of fiber that can cause inflammation of the GI tract. Flax causes constipation because it is very hard to digest. Our guts simply aren't made for consuming flax.

Flax is also a phytoestrogen. Phytoestrogens increase the bad estrogen in your body. Our bodies produce three types of estrogen:

- **Estradiol:** This healthy, or "good," estrogen is produced by the ovaries.
- **Estrone:** Fat cells form and store this unhealthy, or "bad," estrogen.

- **Estriol:** This type of estrogen is produced only in women who are pregnant.

Flax increases estrone, the "bad" estrogen that we don't want. Flax contains more phytoestrogens than any other food, and these phytoestrogens reduce sex drive, increase breast size in men, and increase estrogen-dominant cancers such as thyroid, uterine, ovarian, and breast cancers, as well as prostate cancer in men.

Here is a list of phytoestrogen-containing foods to avoid (in micrograms of phytoestrogens per 100 grams):

- Flaxseed (163,133 mcg)
- Chia seeds (61,055 mcg)
- Soybeans (45,724 mcg)
- Tofu (8,688 mcg)
- Soy milk (7,422 mcg)
- Flax bread (3,770 mcg)

If you find that you are in ketosis but are not losing weight, try eliminating all nuts and nut flours for two weeks. After two weeks, start with ¼ to ½ cup per day of the nuts that are the lowest in total carbs. (Walnuts and macadamia nuts are good options; see Chapter 11 for a complete list of the nuts that are lowest in carbs.) If weight loss stalls or you gain weight (retain water), eliminate nuts and nut flours again for a couple of weeks.

DON'T CONSUME DAIRY

Cut out all dairy, even low-carb, high-fat dairy. Skip the butter, cream, whey protein, cheese, yogurt, cream cheese, and whey protein powder. We find cutting dairy helps many clients more quickly get to their goal weight.

When you have a damaged and inflamed gut, a phenomenon called "atrophy of the villi" occurs. You digest dairy at the ends of the villi, which are little fingerlike projections that line the intestinal wall. If the villi are damaged, you often have a lack of absorption (low ferritin—a blood protein that contains iron—numbers are common in that case), acid reflux, indigestion, gas, and, bloating. Once you heal the intestinal wall with an anti-inflammatory ketogenic diet, you can reincorporate those foods, in smaller amounts at first. We usually have people take healing supplements, such as Zinlori 75 and aloe vera, to rebuild the intestinal wall faster. Egg white protein powder is a good dairy-free substitute for whey protein powder.

If you are in ketosis but are not losing weight or don't feel well, eliminate dairy for two weeks. Weigh yourself the day you start and then weigh yourself again two weeks later. After two weeks, add dairy. Start with ghee or a goat milk cheese to see if your weight plateaus or goes up because you are retaining water. If your weight doesn't rise, try adding another dairy product. If you gain weight after reintroducing dairy (which indicates that you're retaining water), it's a good sign you are still sensitive to dairy.

We recently had a client who added dairy after being in ketosis and eating dairy-free for two weeks. She added ghee and tested well (she didn't gain weight or retain water). The next day, she tried butter and tested well. She added goat milk cheese, then cow milk cheese. Her blood sugars and ketones continued testing well, and she didn't retain water.

Here are some tips for reintroducing and testing with dairy:

- Start with ghee and then try butter.
- Try goat milk cheeses, such as feta.
- Try cow milk cheeses, such as Parmesan.
- Try soft cheeses, such as cream cheese or mascarpone.

 ## DON'T DRINK YOUR CALORIES!

One thing you might not have thought about is that sound is a sensual part of the eating experience. The crunchy sensation we experience is more significant for the sounds it makes inside our heads than it is for how it feels in our mouths. The internal noises of chewing always happen as we eat, but eating a soft omelet is quite different than chewing on nuts or chips, which is one reason why "you can't eat just one."

Our neural sensory systems experience something called *habituation* in which our sensory neurons become less receptive with constant exposure to a stimulus. One reason you might find crunchy foods more appealing lies in the extra engagement of your senses when you eat; you might like a particular food because you like the way it sounds in your head. Chewing crunchy foods not only satisfies your desire for texture but also adds the sense of sound to your eating pleasure.

Drinking calories doesn't signal satisfaction in the brain, and it often leaves us wanting more stimulus, which creates cravings for more food. (This also includes bulletproof coffee, which is coffee mixed with butter, MCT oil, and sometimes heavy cream.) Drinking your calories also doesn't signal the proper hormones, such as leptin and ghrelin, that give you a sense of satisfaction and indicate that you're full as other nutrient-dense whole foods do. Chewing is a powerful tool. Use it! Stick with liquids like water or tea and save the calories for luscious, flavorful foods that you must chew.

BE CAREFUL WITH BULLETPROOF COFFEE

If you consume bulletproof coffee to "fast" until noon, you are no longer fasting. Even if you eat only fat, eating more than 40 to 50 calories takes you out of intermittent fasting. As explained in Chapter 3, consuming only fat will raise insulin enough to stop lipolysis and break your fast.

 ## DON'T EAT IF YOU'RE NOT HUNGRY

Breakfast isn't the most important meal of the day; however, "breaking your fast" is the most important meal of the day! We find that idea that you need to eat every two to three hours to fuel your metabolism and muscles to be ridiculous. Sure, if you are a sugar burner, you need to eat that often, not only because you are "hangry" but also because eating a high-carbohydrate diet burns up amino acids, so you need insulin to increase muscle. However, if you eat a well-formulated ketogenic diet, the protein isn't oxidized, and therefore your muscle is preserved.

Eating breakfast within an hour of waking is not helping your waistline. If you are constantly fueling your body and increasing insulin, you will be shutting off lipolysis (using body fat for fuel), and you will not get into the fat-burning mode. Do not eat every two hours.

A big benefit of intermittent fasting is based on the idea that when insulin is low, lipolysis is enabled and you are burning body fat for fuel! Fat is what most people are trying to get rid of, right? After eight hours, your body is forced to start metabolizing fat.

 ## DON'T DRINK ALCOHOL

We once had a client who told us that he had to have a few glasses of wine in the evening so ketones would be present when he tested his levels in the morning. If he didn't drink the wine, ketones were not present. Our first thought was "Um, what?" Turns out, he was right. A breath ketone tester is a lot like the breathalyzer that police use, and drinking wine before bed can make you register higher ketones in the morning.

When people go on a diet, they often choose the "light" versions of their favorite alcoholic beverages to save a few calories. However, that is only a small piece of the puzzle. After only two alcoholic beverages, fat metabolism is reduced by as much as 73 percent. Oxidative priority forces the body to stop using fat for fuel and start burning alcohol (read more about this in Chapter 3). This scary fact shows that the primary effect of alcohol on the body is not so much how many calories we consume, but how those calories stop the body from using stored fat for energy.

INTROVERTS FIND KETO EASIER TO MANAGE

Are you an introvert or extrovert? Introverts can stick to their diet lifestyles better than extroverts. Why? If you're an extrovert who's always going out with others who do not live the same lifestyle as you, peer pressure often gets the best of you.

WILLPOWER OVER CRAVINGS

If you are having a hard time with cravings, don't blame yourself. Think of willpower as being like a muscle in the brain that can get overworked. You need to limit temptations. You have only a finite amount of willpower to get you through the day, so be careful to conserve it and try to save it for emergencies.

Work and family obligations might require all your willpower, which could lead you to give in to food temptations. We notice that if we stay up too late to work, our minds start to wander to food, and those thoughts can become overwhelming. We know that if we had a pantry filled with junk, we would be tempted to eat it. But we live way out in the country, which makes it hard to run out and get something, and we're not going to turn on the oven to bake late in the evening. Instead, we take L-glutamine to help calm ourselves and our cravings before going to bed. We suggest you do the same.

Here are some more tips to help you stay the course:

- Clean out your pantry of all the junk food. Other people in your house don't need that stuff, either.

- Don't put temptations near you. Just having food where you can see it can deplete your willpower.

- Plan ahead, or cravings, frustrations, and desire can become overwhelming. Make "healthified" brownies and ice cream. We keep these treats in the freezer at all times! We feel a desire to eat sugar- and wheat-filled treats (especially in the summer), but we know that those foods would set us off course. Once you start eating the wrong things, it is a downward spiral!

- Practice. In the short term, self-control is a limited resource. However, over the long term, it can act more like a muscle. Practice, practice, practice equals better willpower. You will gain more control every day.

- Try taking supplements. Supplements such as *Bifidobacteria*, magnesium, and zinc can help with those nasty cravings!

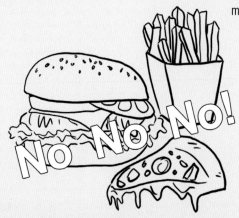

Alcohol Slashes Testosterone Levels

Drinking alcohol is the most efficient way to slash your testosterone levels. A single bout of heavy drinking raises levels of cortisol, the muscle-wasting stress hormone, and decreases testosterone levels for up to twenty-four hours. If you are working out to build strong fat-burning muscles yet are also consuming alcohol, know that this actually breaks down muscle further, and you end up with a slower metabolism as a result. Repairing and building new muscle depends on having the proper hormone levels. If your levels aren't right, your body cannot repair your muscles properly! Women don't want low testosterone levels, either, as testosterone plays a key role in women's reproductive cycles and overall health.

Once ingested, alcohol is converted to a substance called acetate. Unlike a car that uses just one type of fuel, the human body can draw from carbohydrate, fat, and protein for energy. When your blood acetate levels increase, your body uses acetate instead of fat. To make matters worse, the more you drink, the more you tend to eat. Unfortunately, drinking makes your liver work to convert the alcohol to acetate, which means that the foods you consume are converted to extra fat.

If that doesn't sound bad enough, consider the fact that alcohol increases estrogen by up to 300 percent and decreases testosterone levels for up to twenty-four hours. Biochemically, the higher your level of estrogen, the more readily you absorb alcohol and the more slowly you break it down.

Alcohol also affects every organ of the body, with the most dramatic effect being on the liver. The liver cells normally prefer fatty acids as fuel and package excess fatty acids as triglycerides, which they then route to other tissues of the body. However, when alcohol is present, the liver is forced to first metabolize the alcohol (oxidative priority). Because the liver is metabolizing the alcohol, fatty acids accumulate in huge amounts and end up getting stored in fat cells. Excess alcohol permanently changes liver cell structure, which impairs the liver's ability to metabolize fat and causes fatty liver disease.

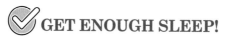 GET ENOUGH SLEEP!

You need eight to ten hours of sleep every night. If you find yourself unable to fall asleep, we suggest taking a cortisol test in the morning and at night (you can buy at-home test kits) to determine whether your cortisol is falling as it should throughout the day. We also suggest getting a ferritin test (a blood test) to determine whether iron is getting into your cells properly. Low iron causes you to feel extremely lethargic, even though you might feel so anxious that you can't sleep.

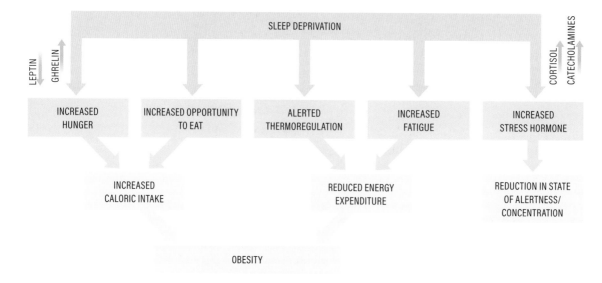

Here are some tips for restful sleep:

- **Enhance your circadian rhythm.** Spend time outside in the sun without UV-filtered sunglasses early in the day to increase serotonin. Wear blue-blocking sunglasses to block blue light from television and electronics later in the day. Blue light inhibits the pineal gland from producing melatonin—our bodies' natural "drowsiness" hormone.

- **Cool down your bedroom.** We open the windows in the winter even when it is –20°F outside. We like to keep our bedroom at around 55°F for sleeping. Keep your room as cold as you can stand to enhance deep sleep.

- **Darken your bedroom.** Try to block out all sources of light.

 SLEEP ISSUES

When I was in my early twenties, I went through a period of terrible sleep issues. Craig started reading to me to help me shut my brain off. Even though I no longer have sleep issues, he still reads to me every night!

- **Rely on white noise.** Add a peaceful noise machine to help block out external noises.
- **Use a grounding mattress or mat.** Adding a grounding mattress or a grounding mat under your sheet can help connect you to the earth and has been shown to help with circadian rhythms and sleep.

If you have trouble falling asleep, do the following one hour before bed:

- **Take magnesium as a natural muscle relaxant.** Try 800 milligrams of magnesium glycinate one hour before bed to help you calm down. Do not buy magnesium oxide; it is not absorbed well and will cause diarrhea.
- **Take one capsule of *Bifidobacteria*.** *Bifidobacteria*, a probiotic, increases serotonin, which in turn increases melatonin production.
- **Take 750 milligrams of GABA.** GABA (gamma-aminobutyric acid) is a nonessential amino acid found mainly in the human brain and eyes. It is considered an inhibitory neurotransmitter, which means it regulates brain and nerve cell activity by inhibiting the number of neurons firing in the brain. GABA is referred to as the "brain's natural calming agent." By inhibiting overstimulation of the brain, GABA promotes relaxation, eases nervous tension, and increases quality sleep. GABA supplements decrease anxiety and emotional eating, improve mood, and shut off "brain chatter" at night; it is nature's Valium.
- **Take 200 milligrams of 5-HTP or 1 gram of L-tryptophan.** The amino acids 5-hydroxytryptophan (5-HTP) and tryptophan increase serotonin, which in turn increases melatonin output. *Note:* Do not take 5-HTP or L-tryptophan if you are on an antidepressant.
- **Use melatonin patches.** Many people say melatonin doesn't work for them, which is most likely due to an absorption issue or leaky gut (the gut isn't absorbing food properly). We suggest a melatonin patch. Absorbing melatonin through the skin works better for many people. Start with 1 milligram and increase as needed.

- **Take pure progesterone.** If you find yourself having a hard time staying asleep and you wake up at 3 a.m. wide awake, the cause is most likely low progesterone (unopposed estrogen) causing estrogen dominance. In this case, we suggest you add a pure progesterone cream, such as Pro-Gest, to an area of thin skin on certain days of your cycle. Many women claim an immediate sense of "calmness" when they apply this to their wrists.

- **Don't eat before bed or exercise at the wrong time of day.** Weight loss is all about fuel supply and demand. With your eating, you have a lot of control over not only insulin but also cortisol and human growth hormone (HGH). Our natural surge of HGH occurs thirty to seventy minutes after we fall asleep, but its antagonist is insulin. If you eat before bed, insulin rises, and HGH, the fat-burning hormone, won't rise because insulin is more powerful. Cortisol is naturally high in the morning and should fall throughout the day. This is why morning exercise is awesome! If you wait until after work to exercise, you'll get another surge of cortisol, which messes with the natural decrease leading up to your bedtime.

ADRENAL FATIGUE

Your adrenal glands are your main stress-adaptation glands. When you are overstressed and your adrenal glands are overworked, your body converts progesterone to adrenal hormones, which depletes you of your anti-anxiety hormone, progesterone. Low progesterone is the leading cause of anxiety, insomnia, and hot flashes.

These are some possible signs of adrenal fatigue:

- Insomnia (you can fall asleep, but wake up many times throughout the night)
- Lack of energy
- Little stressors make you feel anxious
- Low moods
- Low blood pressure
- Bad memory
- Low libido
- Lack of interest in the things you used to love

- Recurring infections
- Asthma or allergies
- The need for coffee or other stimulants for energy
- Hot flashes or PMS
- Loss of menstrual cycle or prolonged cycles

Elevated cortisol uses up tyrosine, an amino acid found in protein that is essential for the thyroid gland to convert from T4 to T3 (the more active thyroid hormone). If there are inadequate thyroid hormones, the adrenal glands are affected; if there are inadequate adrenal hormones, the thyroid doesn't function properly.

The following are some things you can do to limit adrenal fatigue:

- **Decrease stress.** If you hate your job, for example, it's time to find a new one that will fit with your new ketogenic lifestyle. We had a client who quit his job to become a fitness instructor. He looks like a whole new person!

- **Evaluate relationships that are causing too much stress.** Do you have toxic people in your life who are trying to sabotage your health goals? It might be time to find more supportive people.

- **Remember that exercise can be a stressor, too.** Don't plan on running a marathon in the middle of a divorce or shortly after a death in the family. You produce only so much stress hormone each day. During a stressful time, yoga is a better fit. Most of our before-and-after photo testimonies come from clients who are making changes with diet alone—no exercise! Focus on getting your diet right first.

- **Decrease stressful eating situations.** Do you get indigestion or diarrhea after a stressful eating situation such as a lunch meeting? While under stress, your heart rate goes up, your blood pressure rises, and blood is forced away from your digestive system and into your legs, arms, and head for quick thinking. There can be as much as four times less blood flowing to your digestive system, which causes a sluggish metabolism. Even if you're eating nutritious food, you won't be able to properly digest and absorb those nutrients because stress causes a decreased enzymatic output in your intestines. Triglycerides and cholesterol also increase, while healthy gut bacteria decrease. Eating while stressed makes you more susceptible to indigestion, acid reflux, and heartburn. We encourage our clients not to have business meetings over lunch because those meetings can mess with digestion.

- **Cortisol and insulin levels also rise with stress.** Weight loss and health are all about hormone manipulation. When cortisol is consistently raised, you often have difficulty losing weight or building muscle. If cortisol is frequently elevated, belly fat is a common external sign. Belly fat is known as visceral fat (the fat that collects around your internal organs and midsection). Visceral fat is a prominent contributor to the development of diabetes and metabolic syndrome. We suggest that you keep your meetings and lunches separate; try to make lunchtime a peaceful little break from work. Also, try not to eat after an argument. Instead, do some yoga. The blood flow is going to your extremities anyway!

- **Avoid stress.** The adrenal glands are one of the most important organs in the body, yet they are often overlooked by medical professionals. These tiny essential glands secrete sex and stress-response hormones. Internal and external stressors (exercise, lack of sleep, family, work, and the like) have a huge effect on the adrenals and therefore on hormonal (thyroid, progesterone, estrogen, and so on) output. During stressful events, your adrenal glands secrete hormones that help your body respond to the stressors, increase blood sugar, breathing rate, cellular metabolism, and blood flow. Your adrenal glands also produce cortisol, estrogen (men produce estrogen in their adrenals), testosterone, thyroid, and many other hormones—all of which regulate your metabolism, immune system, reproductive system, mineral balance, and excretory functions. People with adrenal fatigue crave salt because they often have low blood pressure. The adrenal glands regulate water and mineral balance in your cells. Without an adequate intake of quality sodium, your blood pressure drops and your adrenals suffer.

TIPS FOR REDUCING STRESS

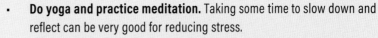

- **Do yoga and practice meditation.** Taking some time to slow down and reflect can be very good for reducing stress.

- **Take a vacation!** There are some striking statistics about Americans not taking vacation time. More than half of Americans don't take all the time off that's allotted them. These workers gave up 658 million unused vacation days in 2016.[3] Vacationing is a great way to reduce stress, recharge your batteries, and enjoy family time or personal downtime. While on vacation, ditch the phone and try to stay disconnected as much as possible. Take time off; you've earned it!

- **Disconnect.** Being connected 24/7 is a symptom of our "always on" modern culture. But always being connected can increase stress. Take some time each day to put your devices away and enjoy a book, get outside, or participate in family activities.

EATING KETO TO HEAL WHILE MAINTAINING OR GAINING WEIGHT

The ketogenic diet isn't just about weight loss. We have many clients who are underweight but still have metabolic syndrome. Sally, for example, weighs 106 pounds, yet she was diagnosed with type 2 diabetes. She doesn't want to lose any weight, but she does need to keep her insulin levels low to help heal her body. How can she accomplish that? We suggested she add more fat calories and increase her protein intake to ensure that she maintains her weight while lowering insulin and reversing her metabolic issues.

chapter 8

Nutrients in a Keto Lifestyle

> I have lost 150 pounds in the last year and a half. My life is so different now. I have a son, [and] after playing with him for 15 minutes I would need to sleep for 2 hours. I had sleep apnea, high blood pressure, my hands would hurt so bad I had trouble holding my phone. I want to thank you for all that you do.

—John

At this point, you might be asking yourself, "If I don't eat fruit and don't eat a lot of vegetables, how will I get my nutrients and vitamins?" The most common criticism of the ketogenic lifestyle is that you can't get all the nutrients your body needs if you don't eat lots of fruits and vegetables. Not only is this a misconception, but there are many other factors that affect nutrient absorption, such as bioavailability, inflammation, and antinutrients.

The source of vitamins and minerals is a really interesting blind spot in most people's view of nutrition, including many doctors and nutrition experts. Ask almost anyone where they get their vitamins and minerals, and fruits and veggies will be the likely answer. We often hear about the latest "superfood" marketing craze (acai berries, goji berries, kale, and the like). As you will see in this chapter, this is mostly marketing hype, not reality, and we hope we can change the perception that you mostly get your nutrients from fruits and vegetables. This chapter might be the most important one in the whole book! We hope we can shift your perspective on which foods you see as nutritious and filled with vitamins and minerals.

We know that nutrient-dense whole foods are the best for our bodies. Your body is looking for nutrients. When you eat foods devoid of nutrients, such as processed foods, you might be eating large volumes of calories, but the calories are not delivering the nutrients your body needs, so you don't get the "I'm full" signal as quickly as you do with nutrient-dense foods.

When it comes to nutrients, though, more is not always better. In most cases, our bodies are very good at removing excess nutrients. However, several factors influence the levels of nutrients our bodies need. One major factor is the type of diet we eat. For instance, when eating a low-inflammation diet, such as a ketogenic diet (low in sugar and omega-6 fatty acids), you have much less need for antioxidants and other nutrients.

The most obvious example is vitamin C. We know that if you don't get enough vitamin C, you can get scurvy. Diets low in fruit are often criticized because you can't get enough vitamin C from meats to prevent scurvy. As it turns out, though, your vitamin C needs are directly affected by your carbohydrate intake. The fewer carbs you eat, the less vitamin C you need.[1] Also, the level of vitamin C needed to prevent scurvy is quite small— about 10 milligrams per day.[2] Contrary to what you will see listed in the nutritional information, there is enough vitamin C in meats to get the 10 milligrams needed to prevent scurvy. According to a study done in 2013, there are about 1.6 milligrams of vitamin C per 100 grams of ox protein.[3] (The amount of vitamin C could be higher because the researchers tested ox protein, not beef or other common proteins.) The USDA labs have a practice of entering 0 grams for vitamin C when testing protein.[4] That means the nutritional info always says 0 grams, even though meat does have vitamin C.

Also, the balance of some nutrients versus other nutrients is more important than the absolute level of each of those nutrients. For example, sodium and potassium are best when in balance. Getting a bit more potassium than sodium might be more important than the absolute sodium level.

Determining the optimal level of micronutrients is difficult because it depends on many factors. However, eating nutrient-dense foods helps you stay satiated and helps ensure that you are getting enough nutrients for the calories you are ingesting. Choosing the most nutrient-dense foods also means that you need fewer calories to get all the nutrients your body needs. It has been shown that eating at a slight caloric deficit leads to a longer life.[5] The most nutrient-dense foods that you can eat might surprise you. Next, we take a look at which foods will give you the most nutrients in every meal.

Our whole family enjoys watching the History Channel television program *Alone.* It starts with ten participants who are placed in the deep wilderness with nothing but a personal video camera. They have to forage for all their food.

The participants who survive the longest in each season share a common theme. They catch fish, but they don't just eat the fish; they also make stock from the whole fish and drink the broth! One participant was unable to catch fish but thrived by trapping mice. He would do a happy dance whenever he trapped one, and then he proceeded to cook it over a fire and eat the whole mouse, bones and all!

Even a vegan participant quickly gave up his dietary lifestyle because he knew he would never survive by spending copious amounts of energy foraging for plants. Being a vegan when you can buy an endless supply of vegetables from a store is one thing, but our ancestors never would have been able to feed whole tribes on plants alone.

My best friend, Laura, was a vegan before she went keto. She tells stories of buying large amounts of food because she was constantly hungry. She says that she thought about food all the time, which distracted her from her work and her personal relationships. She developed a thyroid disorder due to a lack of nutrients, amino acids, and zinc because she never consumed animal protein. Now that she is keto, she eats once a day and thrives on nutrient-dense proteins, and she no longer is plagued by constant thoughts of her next meal.

MEAT, THE REAL SUPERFOOD

Through clever marketing, FDA recommendations, and an irrational fear of meat (due to flawed studies linking the consumption of meat to cancer and other risks), it is commonly thought that fruits and vegetables are the most nutrient-dense foods. Although it's true that some vegetables are high in certain nutrients, if you examine foods critically, you will quickly see that the most nutrient-dense foods are animal proteins such as beef and fish, and that the *real* superfoods are organ meats like liver.

Meats are the best source of complete proteins for building and maintaining muscle and lean mass. But what is seldom talked about is how many nutrients are in meats. The following chart compares nutrients in meats to those found in common foods that are often considered to be "super-fruits" or "super-veggies."

NUTRIENTS IN "SUPERFOODS" COMPARED TO ANIMAL PROTEIN

Per Serving	Apples	Blueberries	Kale	Beef	Beef Liver
Calcium (mg)	9.1	4.5	63.4	11	11
Magnesium (mg)	7.3	4.5	15.0	19	18
Phosphorus (mg)	20.0	9.0	24.6	175	387
Potassium (mg)	163.8	57.8	200.6	370	380
Iron (mg)	0.2	0.2	0.8	3.3	8.8
Zinc (mg)	0.2	0.2	0.2	4.5	4
Selenium (mcg)	0.0	0.1	0.4	14.2	39.7
Vitamin A (IU)	69.2	40.5	13530.9	40	53,400
Vitamin B6 (mg)	0.0	0.1	0.1	0.4	1.1
Vitamin B12 (mcg)	0.0	0.0	0.0	2	11
Vitamin C (mg)	7.3	7.3	36.1	2	27
Vitamin D (IU)	0.0	0.0	0.0	7	19
Vitamin E (mg)	0.2	0.5	0.8	1.7	0.63
Niacin (mg)	0.2	0.3	0.4	4.8	17
Folate (mcg)	0.0	4.5	11.4	6	145

Our Bones Need Fat, Too

The sheaths of our bones primarily are made up of saturated fat. The limited access we've had to saturated fat in our food over the last several decades is one cause of the increase in osteopenia and osteoporosis.

As you can see, animal protein is much more nutrient-dense than these typical fruits and vegetables. And if you want to talk about what is a real superfood, that crown would have to go to offal (organ meats)!

There are many reasons why people don't know that meat is nutrient-dense. Some of those reasons are political, some are simple misconceptions about what is healthy, and others are rooted in corruption. The whole "saturated fat causes heart disease" dogma (described in Chapter 1) was manufactured in large part based on studies funded by the sugar industry. As a result, healthcare and nutrition professionals have shied away from recommending animal proteins and eggs due to their saturated fat and cholesterol content; instead, the recommendation has long been that we limit our intake of those foods. If you aren't getting nutrients from animal proteins and eggs, you need to get it from fruits and vegetables to make up the difference. Fruits and vegetables are the only other nutrient-dense options. As these experts recommended fewer and fewer animal proteins, they recommended more and more fruits and vegetables to compensate. Of course, the addition of more fruits and vegetables just brings more carbohydrates and sugar into the diet, as well as many antinutrients from plant foods (you'll find more on antinutrients later in this chapter).

Let's take a look at a couple more comparisons. The following chart compares nutrients found in common vegetables to those found in beef.

> **Herbs and Spices Are Nutrient-Dense**
> Herbs and spices are some of the most nutrient-dense foods on the planet. Add lots of spices and fresh herbs to make your meals more flavorful and to increase your nutrient intake!

NUTRIENTS IN COMMON VEGETABLES COMPARED TO BEEF AND BEEF LIVER

(Per 100 Grams)	Cauliflower	Broccoli	Kale	Beef	Beef Liver
Calcium (mg)	22	47	72	11	11
Magnesium (mg)	15	20	17	19	18
Phosphorus (mg)	44	66	28	175	387
Potassium (mg)	303	316	228	370	380
Iron (mg)	0.4	0.7	0.9	3.3	8.8
Zinc (mg)	0.3	0.4	0.2	4.5	4
Selenium (mcg)	0.6	2.3	0.5	14.2	39.7
Vitamin A (IU)	13	623	15376	40	53,400
Vitamin B6 (mg)	0.2	0.2	0.1	0.4	1.1
Vitamin B12 (mcg)	0	0	0	2	111
Vitamin C (mg)	46	89	41	2	27
Vitamin D (IU)	0	0	0	7	19
Vitamin E (mg)	0.1	0.8	0.9	1.7	0.63
Niacin (mg)	0.5	0.6	0.5	4.8	17
Folate (mcg)	57	63	13	6	145

Now let's look at fat. Bulletproof coffee and fat bombs are all the rage these days, but what nutrients are you getting by adding all that fat? The next chart illustrates the point that you're not getting much in the way of nutrients.

NUTRIENTS IN COMMON FATS COMPARED TO BEEF AND BEEF LIVER

(Per 100 Grams)	Beef Tallow	Lard	Beef	Beef Liver
Calcium (mg)	0	0	11	11
Magnesium (mg)	0	0	19	18
Phosphorus (mg)	0	0	175	387
Potassium (mg)	0	0	370	380
Iron (mg)	0	0	3.3	8.8
Zinc (mg)	0	0.1	4.5	4
Selenium (mcg)	0.4	0.2	14.2	39.7
Vitamin A (IU)	0	0	40	53,400
Vitamin B6 (mg)	0	0	0.4	1.1
Vitamin B12 (mcg)	0	0	2	11
Vitamin C (mg)	4	0	2	27
Vitamin D (IU)	0	0	7	19
Vitamin E (mg)	5.5	0.6	1.7	0.63
Niacin (mg)	0	0	4.8	17
Folate (mcg)	0	6	6	145

All you're getting are calories and a little vitamin E. This is why some people can drink two bulletproof coffees in a day, which can pack 800 calories or more, but they would struggle to eat thirteen eggs (which is also 800 calories). Chewing helps your body register leptin better to give you that "I'm full" signal, and you get more nutrients from the eggs than you do from just drinking fat. Read more about the difference in drinking calories and eating calories in Chapter 7.

The upshot is that proteins are the real superfoods, and organ meats are the super superfoods. The following figure shows some organ meats and their nutrient contents.

We're not saying you must eat all these organ meats; we're just providing an example of their nutrient content. As you can see, beef liver stands out as one of the most nutrient-dense foods. Other types of liver are great as well. Chicken livers can

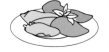

be really tasty fried up in a little oil with some lemon juice and garlic. If you're an adventurous type, try some offal to add a nutrient kick to your diet. When prepared properly,

NUTRIENTS IN OFFAL (ORGAN MEATS)

(Per 100 Grams)	Heart	Tongue	Tripe	Brains	Kidneys	Beef Liver
Calcium (mg)	7	6	69	43	13	11
Magnesium (mg)	21	16	13	13	17	18
Phosphorus (mg)	212	133	64	362	257	387
Potassium (mg)	287	315	67	274	262	380
Iron (mg)	4.3	3	0.6	2.5	4.6	8.8
Zinc (mg)	1.7	2.9	1.4	1	1.9	4
Selenium (mcg)	21.8	9.4	0	21.3	141	39.7
Vitamin A (IU)	0	0	0	147	1397	53,400
Vitamin B6 (mg)	0.3	0.3	0	0.2	0.7	1.1
Vitamin B12 (mcg)	8.5	3.8	1.4	9.5	27.5	111
Vitamin C (mg)	2	3.1	0	10.7	9.4	27
Vitamin D (IU)	trace	0	0	0	32	19
Vitamin E (mg)	0.2	0	0.1	1	0.2	0.63
Niacin (mg)	7.5	4.2	0.9	3.6	8	17
Folate (mcg)	3	7	5	3	98	145

beef tongue can be amazing. Beef tongue tacos, anyone? Kidneys and heart are surprisingly good, too. We love hiding offal in chili. Substitute ground liver for half or a third of the ground beef in the recipe and you won't even notice it.

Animals have a preference for organ meats in the wild. They have an instinct regarding the most nutrient-dense parts of the kill. Carnivores tend to eat organ meats when food is plentiful while skipping the other parts of the animal. For example, Alaskan grizzly bears eat only the salmon brains, skin, and eggs when salmon are plentiful because these are the most nutrient-dense (and fattiest) parts of the fish and are the best for adding weight for the winter hibernation.[6]

Recently, a news story reported that dead great white sharks were washing up on shore with only their livers—and sometimes their hearts as well—missing. It turns out that orcas (killer whales) were attacking the sharks and only eating those nutrient-dense parts.[7] Marine animals are smart and go for the most nutrient-dense options, too!

The following figure shows some of the common proteins (and eggs) we use liberally in a ketogenic lifestyle.

NUTRIENTS IN COMMON KETOGENIC FOODS

(per 100g)	Chicken	Pork	Eggs	Salmon	Beef	Beef Liver
Calcium (mg)	11	5	53	9	11	11
Magnesium (mg)	28	24	12	27	19	18
Phosphorus (mg)	196	296	191	240	175	387
Potassium (mg)	255	489	134	363	370	380
Iron (mg)	0.7	0.4	1.8	0.3	3.3	8.8
Zinc (mg)	0.8	1.4	1.1	0.4	4.5	4
Selenium (mcg)	17.8	40.6	31.7	24	14.2	39.7
Vitamin A (IU)	21	0	487	50	40	53,400
Vitamin B6 (mg)	0.5	0.7	0.1	0.6	0.4	1.1
Vitamin B12 (mcg)	0.4	0.5	1.3	3.2	2	111
Vitamin C (mg)	1.2	0	0	3.9	2	27
Vitamin D (IU)	2	53	35	526	7	19
Vitamin E (mg)	0.1	0.1	1	3.6	1.7	0.63
Niacin (mg)	11.2	8.8	0.1	8.7	4.8	17
Folate (mcg)	4	0	47	26	6	145

As you can see, there is a wider spread now, with the colored units representing the highest and second highest nutrients, which is why a ketogenic diet with lots of nutrient-dense proteins from seafood, beef, pork, poultry, and eggs is a balanced and nutrient-dense diet. Including a variety of ketogenic proteins and eggs in your diet ensures that you get the nutrients you need to thrive.

All these examples show that there is little need to include fruit in your diet because it is not as nutrient-dense as protein and it comes with a load of inflammatory sugar. Eating fruit simply means that you need more antioxidants to combat the inflammation caused by the sugar!

In some instances, vegetables do stack up decently against protein. Although some vegetables come close to offering the same amount of nutrients as proteins, they still aren't as nutrient-dense across all nutrients. Let's take a closer look at vegetables because there are other factors to consider.

GETTING PREBIOTICS FROM MEAT

Are you concerned about not getting prebiotics if you cut out fiber? Did you know that chewing on tasty ribs is a great way to get prebiotics? It is, and so is gnawing on chicken wings, sardines, anchovies, or a fibrous steak! Collagen is the second most effective prebiotic. Call us crazy, but we love to grind up the best cuts of steak into hamburger. Our family eats hamburgers just about every day because marbleized ground beef contains cartilage and connective tissue that is filled with prebiotics!

VEGETABLES AND OUR DIGESTIVE TRACTS

When you eat vegetables, focus on the nonstarchy veggies, such as cucumbers, leafy greens, celery, tomatoes, and peppers. You also need to stop looking at vegetables as superfoods. Animal protein is more nutrient-dense across a wide range of vitamins and minerals, as shown in the previous section. Also, all plants come with antinutrients, the plants' natural defense mechanisms.

Let's start off by looking at vegetables from a biological perspective. If humans are true omnivores, then we should be able to process both protein and vegetables easily. There are two components of the digestive tract that make digesting vegetables possible:

- The first is a larger stomach (proportional to other body parts, such as the brain). Vegetables take up a lot of volume in the digestive tract compared to animal proteins given the amount you need to consume to get enough nutrients.
- The second is the cecum, which is a small pouch in the intestines that is specifically used for digesting fibrous plants. To be properly digested, plant fibers are fermented in the cecum. The following figure shows the human cecum.

THE HUMAN BOWEL

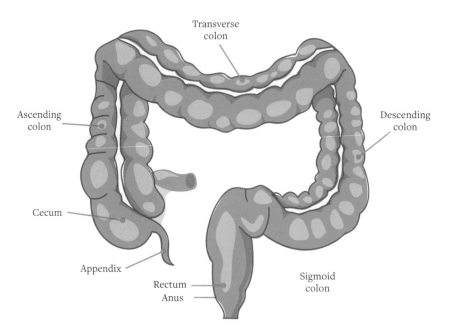

In humans, the cecum is located at the start of the large intestine (that is, at the junction of the small and large intestines). That is why we don't digest fiber and plant material (cellulose) in the same way that true omnivores do. For comparison, a panda's cecum is a very long pouch that can hold a lot of plant material so that it can be fermented before being digested. Humans, on the other hand, have a tiny pouch that can't fully ferment vegetables like true herbivores' ceca. This indicates that humans are intended to be primarily carnivores rather than omnivores. Our theory is that as humans evolved, we developed bigger brains, which required nutrient-dense foods to support and grow. The brain is a fuel and nutrient hog. As our brains grew, our stomachs and ceca shrank. Eating predominantly animal proteins is what enabled this shift to occur. We essentially traded big guts for big brains.

Although humans never fully lost the ability to digest vegetables, they no longer were a primary source of nutrients given the changes in our digestive systems. Based on these evolutionary facts and the fact that veggies are less nutrient-dense than proteins, you can see why veggies are not a primary staple in a ketogenic lifestyle.

VEGETABLES AND ANTINUTRIENTS

Unbeknownst to many people, vegetables contain antinutrients. Each plant has different components, including roots, bulbs, stalk, leaves, and fruit, each of which serves a purpose. However, the fruit is the only part that the plant wants us to eat. If we eat the other components, the plant might die. Let's take a look at a few of those components and the defenses that plants have to prevent us from eating them.

Nightshade plants (potatoes, tomatoes, eggplant, peppers, and others) contain bitter compounds called glycoalkaloids, which are found throughout the plant but concentrated in the leaves, flowers, and unripe fruit. Glycoalkaloids help defend a plant against bacteria, fungi, and some insects—they are natural pesticides. Glycoalkaloids also act as neurotoxins by blocking the enzyme cholinesterase, which is responsible for breaking down acetylcholine. Acetylcholine is a vital neurotransmitter that carries signals between nerve and muscle cells. Research has even shown that too many glycoalkaloids can burst the membranes of red blood cells and mitochondria, which could be a cause of leaky gut.[8]

Cruciferous veggies such as leafy greens (arugula, cabbage, collard greens, watercress, and so on), broccoli, cauliflower, and Brussels sprouts also contain sulforaphane. Sulforaphane is another plant defense mechanism that can kill small insects,

---

Protease Is Necessary to Digest Animal Protein

If you have been a vegetarian or vegan for a year or more, you might find that you feel ill if you try to add animal protein back into your diet. Your body is a brilliant machine; if you don't eat animal protein, your body isn't going to waste energy producing protease, the digestive enzyme that breaks down protein. In this situation, we suggest supplementing with digestive enzymes that contain protease until your body starts to produce protease on its own again. Our bodies also produce fewer digestive enzymes as we age, so we also suggest reintroducing animal protein gradually. Grass-fed bone broth is a great and nutritious food to start with.

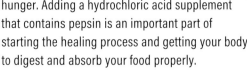

Hydrochloric Acid Supplements

A healthy thyroid produces hydrochloric acid (HCl). If you are low in HCl, you could be eating perfectly but never benefit because you can't absorb nutrients properly. Being low in HCl also increases hunger. Adding a hydrochloric acid supplement that contains pepsin is an important part of starting the healing process and getting your body to digest and absorb your food properly.

bacteria, and worms.[9] It can poison mitochondria and generate reactive oxygen species (ROS, or compounds that promote oxidants and inflammation), among other nasty properties.

When you look at a food—and, more specifically, what is in that food—you have to consider all the components that come with it. Some vegetables are high in certain nutrients but also come with antinutrients, such as glycoalkaloids, that can cause damage. The bioavailability of the nutrients (that is, how readily the body can utilize those nutrients) is important, too. Studies have shown that the phytic acid in foods like legumes and grains can inhibit absorption of nutrients.[10] So the upshot is that maybe those vegetables aren't all good and that we need to take a different perspective when it comes to eating them.

Animal protein is our focus because of its nutrient density and its muscle-building properties. Although our bodies are still able to process some plant material (not the fiber), we must consider the negatives that come with plants and the fact that our biology dictates that, by design, we are mostly meat eaters.

PALEO VEGETABLES

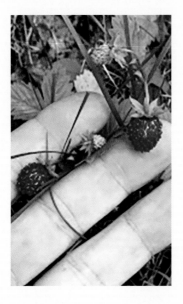

Wild strawberries are tiny compared to their grocery store counterparts.

One last thing to consider when looking at fruits and vegetables is what our Paleo ancestors ate versus what we see in grocery stores today. Almost everything we see in the store today bears little resemblance to what our ancestors ate.

Ancient tomatoes were tiny, maybe ½ inch across. Potatoes were the size of peanuts. Cucumbers were spiny, and lettuce was bitter and prickly. To be edible, peas had to be roasted like chestnuts and then peeled. Beans were naturally laced with cyanide.

The fruits and vegetables available in stores today are fairly recent inventions, and they are the result of years of cultivation and breeding of plants to be bigger, sweeter, and less bitter. In most cases, the emphasis has been on sweetness.

This photo shows a wild strawberry that we found in northern Wisconsin. It is about the size of a pea, and it's quite tart. Can you imagine how long a hunter-gatherer would have to hunt to gather enough of these to equal just one grocery store strawberry?

The breeding of fruits and vegetables is one reason it's impossible to live a true Paleo lifestyle today. None of the fruits and veggies available to us in modern times resemble anything that was available to our hunter-gatherer ancestors. In almost every case, today's fruits and vegetables have been bred to be sweeter, with a higher sugar or starch content, and they almost always have a much lower nutrient density than their Paleo versions.

THE FIBER MYTH

After reading about how humans are designed to be primarily carnivores, you might be asking, "What about fiber? Don't you need lots of fiber to feed your gut flora and keep digestion moving along?" Let's break this down into two components to dispel this myth.

WHAT IS FIBER?

Let's look at our definition of what is or contains fiber. Most people think of plants and vegetables as being sources of fiber. However, once again, we fail to remember that animal products contain fiber, too. Some animal parts, such as connective tissues, contain more fiber than is found in any kind of plant part other than fructo-oligosaccharides (FOS). A diet based mainly on animal proteins can still include appreciable amounts of fiber, especially if you eat sardines, chicken wings, ribs, and so on. Also, you need to consider the other nutrients that come with that fiber. It is likely that the reduction in glucose in the small intestine has far more important health benefits than any of the small effects fiber has on the digestive tract. Look at the following chart. The food highest in fermentable material after FOS is collagen. This means the gut flora can use it for food, which is called a prebiotic.

FOODS WITH THE HIGHEST PREBIOTIC CONTENT

Substrate	Total SCFA
Casein	7.42
Cellulose	1.53
Chicken cartilage	5.50
Collagen	7.96
Fructooligasaccharides	10.37
Glucosamine	7.11
Glucosamine chondroitin	5.36
Rabbit bone	4.14
Rabbit hair	2.18
Rabbit skin	3.36

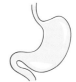

FIBER FOR DIGESTION

The idea that you need fiber to "keep things moving" is also a myth. Adding fiber bulks up your stools, but is that a good thing? It turns out that it isn't. Fiber draws up a lot of moisture and, in most cases, actually makes constipation worse. A study published in 2012 found that stopping fiber improved constipation and associated symptoms.[11] We find this to be true with our clients as well. Clients who stop adding fiber see relief from constipation.

Too much fiber also elongates the intestines, which can cause inflammation and irritation of the bowels. Too much fiber might also contribute to IBS, colitis, colon cancer, and more. The book *Fiber Menace: The Truth About the Leading Role of Fiber in Diet Failure, Constipation, Hemorrhoids, Irritable Bowel Syndrome, Ulcerative Colitis, Crohn's Disease, and Colon Cancer* by Konstantin Monastyrsky discusses the negative effects of fiber consumption in detail.[12]

The "How do I get enough fiber?" question really is irrelevant and likely is contrary to the health benefits it suggests. Eat lots of different animal parts (nose-to-tail eating is best!), and you will get all the prebiotic material you need to feed your gut microbiome.

WHAT ABOUT MEAT AND CANCER?

At this point, you might be asking about the links between red or processed meats and cancer. Let's take a look at these claims and break down why they are not a concern for people following a well-formulated ketogenic diet.

- **Scientific studies:** Let's talk about scientific studies first because they are not all created equal. The devil is always in the details. Who funded the study (see the sugar industry-funded studies in Chapter 1)? What methods were used? What were the confounding factors? The vast majority of studies are fairly meaningless when you account for these factors. However, that doesn't stop the media from blasting news about the latest "red meat causes cancer" study, even though the methods used were flawed and most of the time the relative risk difference was minuscule. For example, let's look at a study that was blasted all over the news with titles like "Eating Meat May Increase Risk of Early Death, Study Finds." First of all, the study cited, titled "Meat Intake and Mortality," was an observational study, which means the creators of the study gave participants a questionnaire asking how often they'd eaten certain foods over the past year.[13] Think about that. How accurately could you describe all the food that you ate in the last twelve months? This lack of control puts any findings into question.

- **Relative risk:** The second thing about this study is that the relative risk (the number of participants affected divided by the number not affected) is only 1.0. In this type of study, anything less than a relative risk of 2.0 really doesn't show a significant correlation.

- **Sourcing and foods eaten with red meat:** Finally, what was eaten with the red meat? Likely a big percentage of the people with a higher red meat intake got that red meat from fast food, which is not the best source of quality meat. It probably came inside a bun, with a side of french fries. They also probably washed it down with a large soda. Was the increased rate of cancer caused by the meat or by everything else that was eaten with the meat?

This is why these types of studies really don't tell you anything.

Another study discussed in a BBC article states that red meat causes death, cancer, and heart risk.[14] Let's compare the two groups used in this observational study to generate these findings about red meat.

Q1 was the group with the lowest red meat intake; Q5 had the highest. Other than red meat intake, what else was different about these two groups that could have resulted in higher rates of cancer and death?

- **Smoking:** Q1 had a smoking rate of 5 percent, and Q5 had a smoking rate of 14.5 percent.

- **Body mass index:** Q1 had an average BMI of 24.7, and Q5 had an average BMI of 26.

- **Physical activity:** Activity (measured in hours) was 27.5 in Q1 and just 17.2 in Q5.

- **Calorie intake:** Total calorie intake was 1,659 for Q1 and 2,396 for Q5.

- **Alcohol consumption:** Q1 drank 8.4 grams of alcohol a day, and Q5 drank 13.4 grams a day.

When you consider all these factors, it is impossible to conclude that the red meat caused the problems. The Q5 group obviously had much less healthy lifestyles, and it was those lifestyles, not red meat consumption, that contributed to the higher rates of cancer and death.

If you aren't looking for something, you aren't going to find it. If you are doing a study to uncover a link between red meat consumption and death rates, you might find an insignificant percentage increase (even though it is likely due to other factors). However, what if the study was looking for a link between sugar intake and death rates? Our guess is that it would result in a many times higher correlation than red meat.

When you read the headlines, be careful to consider the details and make up your own mind about whether the findings of any new study are worth worrying about. We are not worried about our red meat intake.

FINAL THOUGHTS

The vast majority of what we are taught about which foods are best for our bodies is flawed. We hope you now look at fruits, vegetables, and, most importantly, animal proteins in a different light. The fact is that meat has a higher nutrient density and is more bioavailable than any fruit or vegetable. And meat doesn't contain sugar or antinutrients.

We are not saying that you should never eat fruits or veggies. We stick to the fruits that have little or no sugar, such as olives, capers, cucumbers, avocados, and tomatoes. We avoid vegetables with tons of sugar bred into them. We eat some nonstarchy veggies—leafy greens, onions, celery, and cabbage, among others— to add color, flavor, and texture to our meals. You can find a more complete list in Chapter 11.

You need to shift your point of view from eating less meat so that you can eat more vegetables to limiting your vegetable intake so that you can eat more meat. Eating more animal proteins, including organ meats, is where healing with a nutrient-dense diet comes from. We use veggies for their varied hues and textures, not because we think they are adding lots of nutrients. That's why we eat meat.

chapter 9

Fasting

If done properly, fasting can be a great tool for weight loss and healing. There is some confusion about what fasting is, how to do it, and what you can or can't eat and drink while fasting. In this chapter, we hope to clear things up.

Our bodies are uniquely designed to accommodate fasting. In humankind's hunter-gatherer days, fasting—including both intermittent fasting and longer periods of fasting during the lean winter months—was normal. However, fasting has been used in more modern times as well. Here are just a few quotes from historically significant figures:

> 66
>
> *The best of all medicines are rest and fasting.* —Benjamin Franklin
> *The light of the world will illuminate within you when you fast and purify yourself.* —Mahatma Gandhi
> *I fast for greater physical and mental efficiency.* —Plato

When we first heard about intermittent fasting, we thought, "No, no, no. This is not good for anyone who wants to maintain their muscle." However, after diving into what happens when you fast on a well-formulated ketogenic diet, we realized that you do maintain muscle while intermittent fasting, and there are other amazing benefits, too. As we started putting intermittent fasting into practice, we began to experience the physical benefits, and we learned that the mental benefits are outstanding as well!

Intermittent fasting came into our lives almost by accident. With the increased amount of fat we were eating (while also getting adequate protein), we were losing weight and were no longer "hangry." When you are eating the most nutrient-dense foods available, like organic organ meats, quality egg yolks, fresh herbs, and spices, your cells are satiated.

Intermittent fasting is not a diet; instead, it is a way of timing your meals. You can still eat very poorly while practicing intermittent fasting, a decision that will prevent you from reaping as many benefits as you would if you eat a well-formulated ketogenic diet.

EARLY BIRD

I now work and write early in the morning in a fasted state for about three hours, and my mind has never been clearer!

Fasting really isn't as drastic as it sounds. When you sleep, you are beginning to fast a little. During the first ten hours after eating, you are digesting and absorbing nutrients; you don't reach a fasted state until you haven't eaten for more than ten hours. So, if you eat dinner at 6 p.m. and don't eat again until 8 a.m., you will have been in a fasted state for about four hours.

To get the most out of intermittent fasting, we recommend limiting your eating window to eight hours. That means you consume all your calories for the day during an eight-hour period. (Six hours or less is even better.) This includes beverages; only zero-calorie drinks (preferably water) are allowed outside of the eating window. When you go more than twelve hours without eating, you enter a fasted state in which you burn fat more efficiently. So eating all your food within an eight-hour window leaves four hours a day during which your body can get into this beneficial state. If your eating window is only six hours long, your body has six hours to make repairs.

We find it interesting that the mental part of dieting is easy, but the physical part is hard. Knowing you need to cut out carbohydrates is easy, but the physical act of making that change can be tricky. When it comes to fasting, however, the mental aspect is what blocks many of our clients from even trying it. Because fasting sounds impossible, they don't even attempt it! Before we tried it, we thought that, too. We didn't like the idea of fasting—or at least we thought we didn't. We liked eating, but because we were sugar burners, we always wanted to eat. Now that we're both keto-adapted, we save so much time not being plagued by thoughts of food all day.

Fasting is natural for our bodies and, if done correctly, can have therapeutic benefits. In this chapter, we discuss the two main forms of fasting—intermittent fasting and longer, multiday fasting.

INTERMITTENT FASTING

By now, you should understand that inflammation is the true cause of disease and that sugar and starch cause inflammation. However, over-nutrition also can cause inflammation. Numerous studies have shown that periodic fasting can have dramatic results in weight loss and in overall health. An article in *The American*

Water Fast Only

Consuming bone broth while fasting is okay, but we recommend sticking to 1 cup or less during the fasting window. Broth is high in glutamine, which in some people easily turns to sugar in the blood. Many of our clients experience a large increase in ketones and a decrease in blood sugar when they follow our instructions and switch to fasting with water rather than broth. You can drink more broth during your eating window if you like.

Journal of Clinical Nutrition explains numerous benefits to fasting, including improved insulin sensitivity, decreased blood pressure, reduced free-radical damage to cells, and weight loss.[1]

If you think about it, our ancestors didn't have access to an 8 a.m. breakfast, a noon lunch, a 3 p.m. snack, and a 6 p.m. dinner every day; they went through cycles during which food was either abundant or very scarce. This inconsistent availability of food contradicts the idea that your metabolism will slow down and cause you to gain weight if you don't eat five times per day. In fact, intermittent fasting is more effective at reducing insulin resistance than calorie restriction.

We practice intermittent fasting every day. In most cases, we fast for close to twenty hours. For some people, however, this approach is too extreme or doesn't fit their work schedules. In that case, practicing intermittent fasting a few days each week is a great goal. But in the keto lifestyle, intermittent fasting will come naturally over time as you become less hungry throughout the day. Eventually, eating only two meals (or sometimes just one) is exactly what your body needs.

WHY FAST?

The following are a few good reasons to try fasting:

- **Fasting reduces insulin resistance.** Insulin is drastically reduced in a glucagon-dominant state. (Imagine a see-saw; one goes up when the other goes down.) When insulin is reduced, it can't cause inflammation on tissues, which is associated with chronic pain, fibromyalgia, heart disease, asthma, and diabetes.

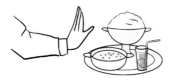

- **Fasting reduces blood pressure.** As your insulin level increases, so does your blood pressure. Insulin stores magnesium, but if your insulin receptors are blunted and your cells grow resistant to insulin, you can't store magnesium, so it passes out of your body through urination. Magnesium in your cells relaxes muscles. If your magnesium level is too low, your blood vessels constrict rather than relax, which raises your blood pressure and decreases your energy level.

- **Fasting reduces triglycerides.** Insulin upregulates lipoprotein lipase (or LPL, a fat-storage promoting enzyme) on fat tissue and inhibits activation of muscle cells. On the other hand, glucagon upregulates LPL in muscle and cardiac tissue while inhibiting activation of LPL in fat tissue.

- **Fasting leads to weight loss.** Eating all your meals in a short window of time typically leads to fewer calories consumed for the day.

- **Fasting reduces cancer.** Fasting cleans out damaged mitochondria, and it "turns on" certain genes that repair specific tissues that would not otherwise be repaired in times of surplus. Intermittent fasting has also been shown to reduce spontaneous cancers in animal studies, which is due to a decrease in oxidative damage or an increase in immune response.

- **Fasting leads to a longer life.** Fasting allows certain cells to live longer (called autophagy, which is the body's process for breaking down old and failing cells and building new ones) because it's energetically less expensive to repair a cell than to divide and create a new one.[2]

So how do you put fasting into practice? There are a lot of ways to do so.

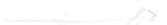

DAILY INTERMITTENT FASTING

Intermittent fasting is a great tool to improve healing, weight loss, and insulin signaling. Intermittent fasting also comes naturally with a ketogenic lifestyle because you aren't hungry all the time.

Compressing your eating window (the time of the day during which you consume calories) really does come naturally for those on a ketogenic diet. Most keto-adapted people find that eating two meals a day works best for them. Whenever you consume calories—regardless of what you eat (fat, protein, or carbs)—your insulin levels rise. A rise in insulin shuts off fat-burning (lipolysis).

The typical American eats three meals spread out through the day, and they also eat snacks between those meals. Eating this way creates constantly elevated insulin levels, which limits the time your body uses fat stores for fuel. The following figure shows the insulin response to a typical day of eating.

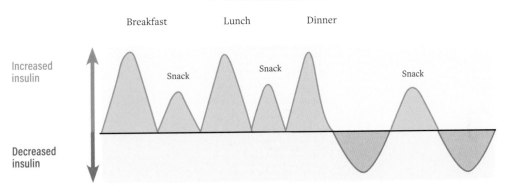

TYPICAL AMERICAN DIET

KETO AND SNACK CONTROL

Intermittent fasting goes beyond how Americans live today. When I ride my bike with my boys, I pass other families and see kids munching on cereal and granola bars—and they aren't even the ones pedaling! I don't want to come off as judgmental, because at one time I was doing the same thing. I was a sugar burner who had to pack snacks if I was going to be away from home for longer than two hours. However, it is so freeing not to have to stop and eat every few hours. If this sounds crazy to you, think about our ancestors. They neither had access to food every few hours nor stopped working to heat food to eat. The microwave has made it too easy for us modern humans, hasn't it?

When you compress your eating window to six hours or less, you are creating a smaller time interval in which insulin is elevated, which makes a much longer timeframe each day during which insulin is low and your body is utilizing stored fat for fuel (lipolysis). The following figure shows the insulin response on an intermittent fasting day.

INTERMITTENT FASTING

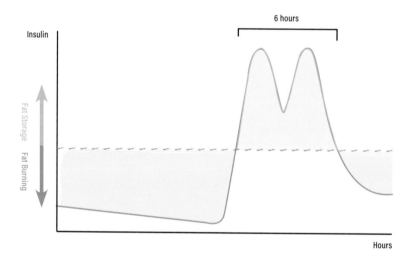

There are several ways to reap the benefits of daily intermittent fasting. Here are a few examples:

- **The morning fast:** The purpose is not to break the human growth hormone and glucagon-dominant state that is called the fasted state. The morning fast works best for people who do cardio in the morning or afternoon. Morning fasts keep the fat-burning hormone (human growth hormone) high. When you eat, insulin rises, which pushes human growth hormone down. Your body gets energy from food sources (calories) or body stores (glycogen, body fat, and muscle). If you want to burn sugar, go ahead and eat before your workout; if you want to burn fat, skip eating beforehand and work out in a fasted state. During the morning fast, use the following guidelines:
  1. You can have coffee if you don't have anxiety, adrenal fatigue, or a thyroid disorder.
  2. You can drink tea and water.

3. For the most benefits, don't consume any calories during the fasting window. However, anything less than 40 to 50 total calories generally will not totally break the fast.

4. We recommend you take amino acids, such as L-carnitine, upon waking (try 3,000 milligrams). Amino acids help shuttle triglycerides to the mitochondria where fat is burned.

- **The evening fast:** If you aren't exercising, we prefer evening fasts because they keep you from bingeing later in the evening. Eat breakfast and lunch; then fast until the next morning.

- **A combination:** Intermittent fasting should last at least eight waking hours. One way to accomplish this is to have dinner no later than 3 p.m. For example, if you go to bed at 10 p.m. and wake up at 6 a.m., you would consume only calorie-free liquids, such as water, green tea, or coffee (decaf if you have adrenal or hormone issues), after waking. We suggest taking L-carnitine first thing in the morning. We then recommend doing cardio (we like to run from 7:30 to 8:30 a.m.). Break your fast at 9 or 10 a.m. This approach leaves a total of eighteen hours between meals, with you being awake for ten of those hours.

Regardless of which method you choose, make sure to stop eating at least three hours before bed because eating later in the evening can lead to weight gain and impaired fat metabolism.[3] That means no calories at least three hours before you go to sleep.

There are a lot of ways to add fasting into your life. For one, we suggest skipping dinner once or twice a week. Maybe you choose a day you know you will get home late and will be eating too close to bedtime. We like this plan because it stimulates human growth hormone to be at a high level when you fall asleep. Some clients are so fat-adapted that they do this every day by not eating after 3 p.m. Skipping dinner takes some adjustment; it's easy when you are a fat-burner, but if you are a sugar-burner and you continue to have a "treat" of sugar or carbs every once in a while, it is a hard thing to practice. Clients who are fat-burners have emailed us to say that they no longer wake up hungry (or should we say, "hangry").

SARCOPENIA

There is a phenomenon called *sarcopenia* in which we lose 1 percent of our muscle mass per year starting at age 25. When you skimp on protein, your body needs amino acids to function properly, so it takes the protein from your healthy muscles to get it, which is not good! Make sure to get enough protein.

INTERMITTENT FASTING WHILE STILL ENJOYING FAMILY TIME

Often, our clients tell us that they can't eat dinner earlier than 8 p.m. because their kids participate in activities in the evening, which leads them to snack at 5 p.m. to make it to a late dinner. We tell them to eat their own dinner earlier and to feed their children later.

We have the opportunity to work with a variety of doctors. When we asked a psychologist about the importance of family dinners and whether eating together is really that significant, he said that it isn't the act of eating that keeps families together. Instead, spending time together is what's important.

We eat our last meal way earlier than our kids do, but we spend quality time preparing keto foods, riding bikes, and fishing—all together. We find family time outside of mealtime. Think about it: At meals, you are usually focused on chewing rather than talking anyway. You can practice intermittent fasting while finding quality family time elsewhere. Our fondest memories are of the conversations we have with the boys while fishing in the afternoons.

Fasting is a very natural process for our bodies. Our hunter gatherer-ancestors didn't have refrigerators stocked with snacks that they ate all day. They would capture an animal, have a feast, and then fast for some time until they were able to get more food. Food came in bursts.

Give fasting a try. Implementing intermittent fasting might be easier after you are keto-adapted, meaning it could be challenging in the first week or so of becoming keto-adapted. However, after a week or two of being keto-adapted, fasting is easy and natural on a well-formulated ketogenic diet!

LONGER FASTS ALLOW APOPTOSIS TO OCCUR

Fasting can be beneficial if done correctly. If you are following a well-formulated ketogenic diet, fasting can be natural and easy to do because you aren't hungry very often. Daily intermittent fasting is especially easy because you just aren't as hungry throughout the day, which makes compressing the eating window easy.

Longer fasts are a more therapeutic form of fasting. They enable your body to perform repair activities when it no longer must worry about digestion. A process known as apoptosis increases when longer fasts are done correctly. Apoptosis—or programmed cell death—is the body's process for killing bad, old, or failing cells.

Your body doesn't kill cells willy-nilly; it is smart, and it isn't going to kill healthy cells. The process of apoptosis goes after the failing, aging, and diseased cells first. Apoptosis is a powerful tool for reversing aging and disease.

There has been evidence to show that fasting helps with cancer. Both intermittent and longer fasts can be beneficial. One study showed that fasting during chemotherapy reduced the side effects and helped protect healthy cells against the therapy.[4] This has led some to quip, "What is helping more, the chemo or the fasting the chemo induces because the patient can't keep food down?"

There have even been amazing restorative examples of long-term fasting when it is done correctly. This person, under supervision, did three- to five-day, water-only fasts each week for six months:

I did short three- to five-day fasts weekly for six months for a terminal heart condition. It did break down muscle mass! My heart went from enlarged and stiff to high-normal size and flexible. I fasted well, and I feasted well! My terminal heart condition is no longer terminal! My cardiologist is amazed!

The increased apoptosis breaks down the aging and diseased heart cells. Proper refeeding builds up new, younger, and healthier cells. This example shows the power of fasting when done correctly, but this intensive form of a fasting treatment should only be done under medical supervision.

When doing a proper long-term, water-only fast, you do not take in any calories. You want to get into a state in which your body doesn't have to use any energy for digestion and can focus all of its energy on repair. You should add electrolytes (4 grams of sodium and 4 to 4.5 grams of potassium) for the first couple days of this water-only fast. You might be able to take just potassium because it is the more important of the two, but taking both should be fine. It depends on your electrolyte levels and your state of ketosis. You shouldn't take only sodium because doing so can keep glucose high and hinder your results. After the second or third day, you can reduce the sodium and potassium because your body will have begun to preserve potassium and derive more potassium from the lean tissue it is breaking down. After all, as explained in Chapter 8, protein contains a lot of potassium, so once apoptosis kicks in at a higher level, less supplemental potassium is needed.

The real magic of apoptosis starts to kick in when your glucose levels fall below your ketone levels (in millimoles, or mmol). This drop usually happens around the fifth day of a water-only fast. For example, blood glucose could drop to maybe 3.3 mmol (60 mg/dL), and ketones could rise to 4 mmol. When your ketones are higher than your blood glucose, you are in a deep state of fasting, and apoptosis ramps up. The following chart shows how apoptosis increases during a longer fast.

For the first two or three days of a seven-day fast, add electrolytes (sodium, potassium, and magnesium). On days 4 and 5, glucose dips below ketones and apoptosis ramps up. After the fast, refeed with lots of protein.

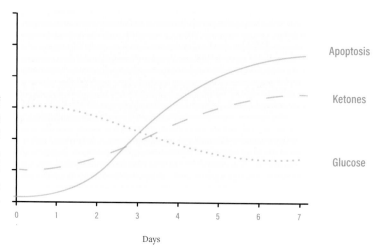

PROTEIN-SPARING MODIFIED FAST

A protein-sparing modified fast (PSMF) is another form of fasting that can be very helpful. Be sure to read about it Chapter 4. This modification doesn't give you as many of the benefits of a water-only fast (such as apoptosis), but it does give you fat-burning benefits while preventing losses of lean mass.

Most people who don't have a chronic disease should do a five- to seven-day water-only fast once or twice a year. One or two such fasts are all most of us need to reap age-reversing benefits. Those with chronic disease might need to go to a more therapeutic level of fasting or do longer or more frequent fasts under medical supervision.

The second component of a proper long fast (that is, a fast of more than twenty-four hours) is to immediately follow it with a proper refeeding. If you did the fast properly and your body killed off and removed aging and failing cells, you should rebuild that lean mass right away. You should exceed your normal protein goal for a few days, which gives your body lots of substrate (amino acids) to rebuild the lean mass that was lost.

One of the worst things you can do is switch to a low-protein diet after a longer fast. During the fast, your body breaks down a bunch of lean mass but doesn't have enough protein to rebuild it, resulting in less lean mass. Loss of muscle mass is not good for long-term health.

For the first four to seven days after a longer fast, we suggest eating at least 1.0 times your lean mass in protein each day. Then you can go back to your normal protein target of 0.8 times your lean mass (as described in Chapter 4).

Fasting is natural for our bodies, and it can be therapeutic if done properly. So fast well and refeed properly.

MORNING PEOPLE HAVE AN EASIER TIME WITH FASTING

Maria is thankful that she's always been a morning person. We see clients who are night owls and find fasting very challenging. When you stay up too late, hunger can get to you, and your mind thinks overwhelmingly of food—and not typically of food that falls into the pure protein and fat categories. Instead, night owls often think about potato chips or ice cream, which is why you shouldn't keep this stuff in the house for anyone! Your kids, spouse, or housemates don't need that junk, either.

chapter 10

Exercise and Keto Athletes

We were both overweight when we fell in love. We joke that we gained "love weight"! We went out for bagels and mochas for breakfast, made sandwiches for lunch, and ate pizza for dinner.

We both had a lot of weight to lose, and we chose different paths when it came to exercise. We live very different lives when it comes to activity. Can you guess who reads higher ketones, even though we both eat the same foods?

Maria rarely sits down. Even while writing, she runs on a trail in the woods. No lie. She often works and answers emails on a run. (We don't recommend this, though, because Maria has tripped and cracked her phone a few times while working and running at the same time.) The point is that Maria loves movement; she craves it. If she's not running, she's kayaking, riding bikes with our kids, swimming, or jumping off the dock. Exercise is Maria's natural antidepressant. However, because of her constant movement, Maria's ketones are low. (We explain more about this soon.)

Craig is the scientist in our partnership. He spends most of his time researching the latest science and talking to the top doctors who specialize in the keto diet, as well as creating websites, meal planners, and macro calculators. Not only is he brilliant at understanding the physics of how things work, but he is a master at breaking information down so that even someone who has never heard of ketosis can understand it. Anyway, he prefers to spend his time working at the computer and sometimes builds things like treehouses for our boys.

The point is that we move our bodies very differently, and this affects our ketones tremendously. Is it a bad thing that Maria's ketones are so low? No. You need to stop chasing high ketone numbers because they don't matter; results are what matter. Adding enough fat even to high-carb items will increase ketones. For instance, you could eat a huge bowl of rice or sweet potatoes and dump MCT oil over the dish (something we don't recommend doing), and you will read ketones when testing. Will you be in lipolysis? Nope. Your ketone numbers do not matter—at all!

If you are an exercise fanatic and are upset that you do not read high ketones, you need to understand that you are utilizing your ketones for your exercise so there will be fewer ketones in your blood. This isn't a bad thing. Stop stressing about testing; instead, focus on your results and how you feel. Do not add more

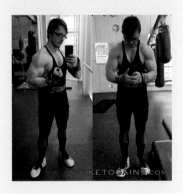

fat just to read higher ketones because doing so will prevent you from burning body fat. There is no need to utilize body fat to make ketones if you keep consuming excess dietary fat.

Exercise is more about building mitochondria than burning extra calories. Mitochondria are the powerhouse part of our cells in which fat is oxidized. The more mitochondria you have and the healthier they are, the more fat oxidation that takes place. Many things are deadly to mitochondria, such as poor diet, aspartame, and many medications, such as the statin drugs that are used for lowering cholesterol. Having healthy mitochondria is one of the keys to longevity, and exercise is one of the best ways to ensure that you have lots of healthy mitochondria.

COMMON MYTHS

In this section, we debunk some common myths regarding ketosis and athletes.

MYTH: YOU NEED CARBOHYDRATES TO BUILD MUSCLE

Keto-adapted athletes have a much higher fat oxidation rate than athletes who are consuming a carbohydrate-rich diet, which is advantageous because glycogen stores are depleted much faster than fat stores. Consequently, keto-adapted athletes using fat for fuel have the aptitude to work out for much longer than their carb-loading competitors.

How to Build Muscle

- **Eat sufficient protein.** Eat between 0.8 and 1.2 grams of protein per pound of lean mass, depending on your activity level and goals. To increase muscle, you need additional energy from calories, primarily protein. You can't build muscle from sweat alone. Calories from protein are better utilized because it aids in muscle growth and repair. Also remember that if you are eating keto, your body fat is a "safeguard," which is why many athletes still can build muscle even while in a caloric deficit as long as they are getting adequate protein.

CARB-FREE MUSCLE BUILDING

Think you can't build muscle without carbs? Check out Luis from KetoGains:

"I have been practically eating one meal per day for a year, ranging between 1,300 to 1,900 kcals—with adequate nutrient partitioning and whole foods. No binges/cravings outside of the usual."

—Luis Villasenor

JUST ME AND MY ELLIPTICAL

When I was in college, I didn't feel like I fit in. I was twenty, married, and didn't feel comfortable in my skin. I purchased a high-performance elliptical machine. Craig traveled often for work, and I ended up spending hours a day watching television and studying while gliding away on my machine in a desperate attempt to lose weight. I spent so much time on that machine that I even ate while working out! No lie! I would get hungry during my workouts, so I would eat.

Of course I was hungry! I was eating nothing but carbs. I considered myself to be an athlete, and in my nutrition classes we were taught you need seven to eleven servings of whole grains to fuel your body. I'm so embarrassed to tell you that I ate a bag of baked potato chips (cheddar flavor) and dipped them in ketchup while on my elliptical! Seriously. I must have looked so ridiculous. However, I was desperate. My exercise and low-fat, low-calorie eating were supposed to help me lose weight, but they never did.

The elliptical machine that I purchased was top-of-the-line. It was meant for gyms where it would get hours of use a day. I would watch a whole Packers football game—beginning to end—while gliding away. I exercised on the elliptical machine so much I broke the ball bearing on it. When I brought it in to get fixed, the guy asked how many people were using the machine. I told him just me. He said, "That's impressive, because a top-notch machine like this can withstand hours of use at a gym."

Because I was in a state of overtraining, I started having trouble sleeping at night. I believe the food I was eating kept me in a state of depression. I never wanted to leave the house, and I now know how detrimental that was to my health. I needed sunlight, grounding, and fresh air! I was too afraid of my own shadow, I was not confident, and I just waited until my love Craig would come home from his work travels. I was so shy that when I had the opportunity to travel with Craig for his work to Germany, I barely left the dreary hotel room. He worked long hours at a trade show, and I sat in my room on Thanksgiving watching National Lampoon's Christmas Vacation. I am not the same person I was then. Now, I would be gallivanting around Munich, exploring every nook and cranny! However, the food I was eating then kept me in a low-dopamine state of depression.

I am opening up to you like this because eating keto has changed me, and it can change you, too! Do not waste your life as I did! You deserve to be the confident and amazing person you were destined to be! Don't let food keep you down.

By the way, I am writing this while floating down a beautiful river in my kayak. I make an effort to make every day special now. I usually work and write while enjoying nature. Even when I lift weights, I refuse to go to the gym because it is nothing but fluorescent lights, and I never enjoy it. I work out outside in nature. I save time by not driving to the gym, and I save money on a gym membership!

- **Strength train!** When you overload your muscles progressively, strength training stimulates muscle growth and causes muscle hypertrophy (enlargement of muscle cell size).
- **Rest.** Your muscles break down as you lift, and they repair as you rest. Getting good sleep is important for human growth hormone (HGH) production at night and repairing and building new muscle.
- **Repeat.** Eat keto, strength train, and rest. Objects in motion stay in motion. Do not get derailed by peer pressure to do carb-ups or drink alcohol. Good habits build great bodies.

MYTH: YOU NEED A LOT OF CARBS IF YOU'RE THIN

We get frustrated when people tell us they eat a lot of carbs and stay skinny or that their spouses won't eat keto with them because they are skinny and can eat whatever they want.

We have a twenty-eight-year-old client who lives in Hawaii, and recently she had her first baby. We consulted with her numerous times last year. Her A1c was 11.4, and she was having strokes! She wanted to live to see her baby girl grow up, so she knew she had to change.

Within six months, we got her A1c down to 4.6, which is incredible! However, she contacted us again recently and said she wished she would gain weight when she cheated because that would help her stay on the diet! We are a vain society, which leads us to change things when we realize that we look bad.

No matter how she looked on the outside, this client needed to heal the internal inflammation. No one saw her unhealthy body (she had inflamed fat cells but didn't have a lot of them). No one judged her for what was in her shopping cart. She didn't take up two seats on an airplane like some obese people. However, she was just as unhealthy as an obese type 2 diabetic.

We often work with clients who have Alzheimer's disease, and they are often very thin. Alzheimer's is sometimes known as type 3 diabetes because the brain is no longer able to use glucose properly.

Just because you are not overweight doesn't mean that you can't get the wonderful benefits that a keto-adapted life has to offer. Our whole family has benefited, and we will never, ever go back!

_#

GIVE KETO A CHANCE

I did a radio interview, and after I finished I continued to listen to the broadcast. The interviewer mentioned that everyone has a different body type and talked about a friend who could eat huge roast beef sandwiches on massive baguettes but remained thin as a rail. I had already left the studio, but I was so upset; I wanted to tell the interviewer about our many clients who are thin but have diabetes. As discussed in Chapter 2, you can have a small number of fat cells that are overstuffed and have diabetes as a result, even if you are thin. We call the phenomenon of skinny people with diabetes the Asian Paradox because many Asians eat a lot of rice and stay thin. However, Asia has a huge type 2 diabetes epidemic.[1]

Is keto the way to eat for everyone? We get this question often, and we do believe everyone can see benefits. After my radio interview, the next woman who was interviewed was a Paleo consultant who claimed she had tried keto but had added rice and some fruit because she feels better when she eats carbs. ARGH! I wished I had still been there so I could have told that woman she likely was dehydrated, which causes lethargy and low moods in the first few weeks of becoming keto-adapted. She needed more salt and electrolytes in the beginning stages (see pages 80 to 86) because carbs were no longer retaining water for her.

MYTH: YOU NEED CARBOHYDRATES FOR FUEL

We also find it to be narrow-minded when an athlete says he or she needs carbs for fuel. If you believe this, we urge you to read the following:

- **Our bodies store more than 40,000 calories as fat, but we can store only 2,000 calories of carbs.** This limited carb storage is why carb-burning marathoners "hit the wall" and constantly need gel packs (containing carbs and potassium) and sports drinks, yet still are low in performance at the end of races because of the depletion of carbs in their muscles and liver. They've used up the available glucose for fuel.

- **Carb-ups and sugar-based fuel sources create a body that fuels on carbs while simultaneously inhibiting fat burning.** After a carb-up, lipolysis is inhibited for days—not just during the hours immediately following the carb-up. You can't switch from carb-burning to ketosis quickly. It takes two to four weeks to adapt fully.

- **You have only 2,000 calories of glucose storage for energy yet you have more than 40,000 calories of fat for energy.** Even athletes who have very little body fat can work out twenty times longer at their maximum level. Vigorous exercise fueled on carbs depletes an athlete in a few hours, but when you are burning fat for fuel, you can exercise for days. Ketosis is great for athletic performance. Our bodies can store more than 40,000 calories (even in lean athletes) of fat but only 2,000 calories of carbs, so when we're burning fat instead of sugar, there's a lot more fuel available at any given time. Consider that migratory birds and whales rely on stored fat to fuel their journeys; they are fat burners. Developing your fat engine increases the amount of energy you can generate and reduces the amount of carbohydrate you use. When combined, you have a more stable and enduring energy supply, better endurance, and faster finish times.

USING EXERCISE EFFECTIVELY IN A KETOGENIC LIFESTYLE

Maria loves weight lifting—for herself and for our clients. For example, one of our male clients was fifty-seven years old and was training for a triathlon. When he started a very low-carb diet, he weighed 180 pounds and had a BMI of 25. After the first two weeks (during which his training intensity was decreased), he said he had the best training and energy of his life! In only twelve weeks, he lost 23 pounds of fat and gained 6 pounds of muscle!

MYTH: YOU NEED TO EXERCISE TO LOSE WEIGHT

Many people gain weight when training for marathons. If you believe the "eat less and exercise more" myth, remember that it takes 3,500 calories to burn a pound of fat. That would require running a marathon and a half! It's not realistic to not eat on the day you run a marathon simply to burn one measly pound of fat.

There is more going on when you exercise. Exercise is a stressor. It can be a good stressor, but in excess it can cause your adrenals to go into overdrive, which increases insulin and results in an inability to lose weight. As you exercise, your insulin goes up, and your hunger goes down. However, it often causes a deeper low in blood sugar, causing you to be hungrier.

When we want to lose weight, we sometimes focus on the number on the scale and forget about the importance of losing body fat. The majority of body fat (more than 80 percent) is stored in fat cells. To get rid of that fat, you need to burn it for energy. You need to get into a negative fat flux (or a negative fat balance), where you are burning more fat off your body than you are taking in through your diet.

When your body is accustomed to burning fat for fuel, it can use body fat as well as dietary fat, which makes keto a great way to lose weight. When you increase the amount of energy your body needs by exercising—and you don't increase your dietary fat—almost all that extra energy comes from burning body fat! However, if you are a sugar burner and you fuel your body with carbs, you burn mostly sugar instead, making it much harder to lose body fat.

We have found that about 80 percent of losing weight is getting the diet right. When the diet is right, you start tapping stored body fat for fuel, which enables you to start losing body fat. Exercise can also help, but it is more important to get the diet right first. You can't exercise enough to compensate for a bad diet.

Next, let's take a look at some of the most effective kinds of exercise and our tips for getting the best results from each one.

CARDIO

Awesome things happen to your body when you work out at an intense rate. Not only does cardiovascular exercise improve the efficiency of your heart and lungs, but it also increases the rate at which your body burns fuel. Over time, burning more fuel means that you will lose weight.

I know that those of you who are fans of Gary Taubes, author of *Why We Get Fat: And What to Do About It,* will think we are wrong. Taubes believes that exercise has nothing to do with weight loss. We understand his points, but we have seen the benefits of exercise and cardio, especially when it comes to losing body fat. Many metabolic changes occur with cardiovascular exercise that uniquely enhances fat metabolism, including the following:

> ### A Moderate Increase in Insulin = a Significant Decline in Fat Loss
>
> Fat loss or lipolysis is significantly lowered with a moderate increase in insulin. Something like a banana elevates insulin for a longer period, leaving less time to burn body fat for fuel. Is a banana "the devil"? No, but it will halt your efforts to burn fat. And, as explained in Chapter 8, you don't need the banana. You can get all the nutrients you need from eating animal proteins that don't come with sugar.

- **A major boost in the number and size of mitochondria.** These parts of a cell are the only places where fat is burned and oxidized. They are the cell's fat-burning furnaces. Having more mitochondria that are healthier increases the amount of fat you can burn.

- **Increased oxidative enzymes.** Cardio exercise causes an increase in the oxidative enzymes that speed up the transport of fatty acid molecules to be used for energy during cardiovascular exercise. (In other words, fat gets to the mitochondria faster, so the body can use it for fuel during exercise.)

- **Increased oxygen delivery through blood flow.** Cardio improves oxygen delivery via blood flow, which helps cells oxidize and burn fat more proficiently.

- **Increased epinephrine sensitivity.** Cardio amplifies the sensitivity of muscles and fat cells to epinephrine, which helps increase the release of triglycerides into the blood and the muscles so they can be burned as fuel.

- **Faster movement of fatty acids into muscle cells.** Cardio creates an increase in the rates at which specialized protein transporters move fatty acids into the muscle cells, making fat more readily available for energy.

- **More fatty acids are allowed into the muscle.** Cardio boosts the amount of fatty acids allowed into your muscles, which also makes fat more readily available for energy.

Pumping Iron

Iron is needed to carry oxygen to the mitochondria of your cells, where fat is burned during oxidation. (As you might guess from the names, oxidation requires oxygen.) An iron deficiency means that your body has a more difficult time burning fat. Worse, when you push yourself too hard, you end up depleting this mineral even further. If you are a woman and you feel tired, are losing hair, and not losing weight with exercise, you are likely low in iron. About 90 percent of women who are low in iron can attribute the deficiency to three causes: menstruation (loss of blood equals loss of iron); a gluten-filled diet, which inhibits the body's ability to absorb iron; and/or excess cardio.

With consistent, progressive cardiovascular exercise, we can truly expand our bodies to be awesome fat burners. When our bodies are tired, and we want to stop exercising, it's gratifying to know that when we push through the pain, we are creating more fat-burning furnaces (mitochondria)!

STRENGTH TRAINING

Most women choose cardiovascular or aerobic exercise, and Maria used to be one of them. She would run 12 miles a day and compete in marathons, but the scale didn't budge. When she finally started taking a fitness class called BodyPump, which uses light to moderate weights, the pounds began to melt off.

Aside from weight loss, there are other benefits to strength training:

- **Improved mood:** Strength training helps lift your mood. Studies prove that watching yourself lift heavier and heavier weights builds confidence and reduces depression, even if you aren't losing weight.
- **Healthy bones:** Strength training builds healthy bones.
- **Stronger and healthier body:** Strength training helps you develop a strong and healthy body for daily movement throughout life.

Multi-joint exercises are the most beneficial movements because they use more than one muscle in a single movement. For example, the bench press works both the shoulder and the elbow joints as well as several muscle groups. Your metabolism and heart rate are directly related to the total volume of muscle mass being used, so multi-joint movements burn more calories by stimulating more muscles.

Some people are concerned that a low-carb diet, like the ketogenic diet, will prevent them from building muscle with strength training. However, in a well-designed low-carb, high-fat diet, there is less protein oxidation and double the fat oxidation, which means muscle is preserved while you burn fat! Muscle is built with protein, not carbs or fat.

There are a lot of myths floating around about strength training. Let's take the top myths down one by one.

Myth: Cardio Exercise Is Necessary for Weight Loss

Although cardio exercise is important, it isn't the only type of exercise that can help you lose fat. Strength training increases muscle mass, and the more muscle you have, the more calories you'll burn all day long (increased basal metabolic rate as muscle expends more energy all day long).

Muscle is denser than fat and takes up less space. That means when you lose fat and gain muscle, you'll be slimmer and trimmer.

Myth: Lighter Weights and More Reps Tone Muscle

To create strong muscles, you must lift enough weight to break down the muscles so they can be repaired to be even stronger. Muscles break down as you lift, and they repair and grow as you rest. If you plan on doing fifteen triceps curls, lift a weight that allows you only to do fifteen curls. You want your body to feel the difficulty of lifting the weight so that the muscle becomes defined. That lean, defined look comes from losing body fat. Heavy weights equal more fat-burning!

Myth: Strength Training Makes Women Bulk Up

This myth persists regardless of the fact that women don't have the amount of testosterone required to build huge muscles. In fact, even men struggle to gain muscle; they have to spend hours lifting to create a muscular physique.

THEY CALLED ME THUNDER THIGHS

When I was a kid, my nickname was Thunder Thighs. My older sister gave me this nickname, and it stuck with me until adulthood.

At the time, I despised her for her cruelty. However, as I look back, I now know that being hurt forms us into strong butterflies. I also now know that people who hurt you like that generally aren't comfortable in their own skin. It's all about them and not about you. My sister and I had the same body type, so clearly she wasn't comfortable in her skin.

You might think it's weird for me to be grateful for what my sister said to me, but I am because it formed me into the strong, compassionate woman I am today. When I was younger, I was afraid of lifting and squatting heavy weights because I thought it would make my thighs even bigger! However, when I started lifting heavy weights and eating keto, my body shape transformed. I stopped being a cardio queen and embraced my strong thighs!

Are You Gaining Weight with Strength Training?

One reason women say their pants fit tighter after lifting heavier weights is that they are overconsuming carbohydrates. Don't grab oatmeal and skim milk—or worse, a brownie—after all your hard work. Did you know that a pound of fat is 3,500 calories, and running a whole marathon burns only about 2,500 calories? Don't think that just because you performed a kick-butt workout, you can reward yourself with a bag of candy. Learn the proper ways to fuel your body because it's essential for your health and outward appearance. And treat yourself in other ways! A one-hour massage is a great way to reward your muscles for their hard work.

Lifting heavy weights can benefit both men and women. Challenging your body with heavy weights is the only way you'll really see results and get stronger. Maria has been lifting heavy weights for years, and she has never even come close to looking like a bodybuilder. Most women who lift weights regularly would agree. Remember, muscle takes up less space than fat. Adding muscle (along with doing cardio exercise and a eating healthy diet, of course) helps you lose fat, which means that you'll be leaner and more defined.

INTERVAL TRAINING

Interval training is basically what it sounds like—alternating intervals of high-intensity and low-intensity exercise. It's based on a simple concept: go fast, go slow, and repeat. This concept sounds simple, but this formula has an incredible number of potential variations and strategies.

Interval training is our favorite way to burn the most calories possible. Not only do you burn a ton of calories while you're doing it, but it also stimulates your metabolism to a far greater degree than lower-intensity training. This is referred to as the *afterburn effect*.

Interval training causes your muscles to go crazy with activity; think of it as a metabolic disturbance. This crazy metabolism boost causes lots of calorie-burning that occurs after exercise to get your body back to normal. The result is that you end up burning more fat and calories in the post-exercise period as your body tries to get things under control.

Here are the basics of interval training:

1. To begin, start your workout at an easy pace and slowly increase your heart rate for at least five minutes. You can use a heart rate monitor or just use a "rate of perceived exertion" test to judge how hard your workout is on a scale of one to ten. A one is resting; a ten means you are working as hard as possible.

2. When you're warmed up, you're ready for an explosion of high-intensity work. Break into a jog or sprint, depending on what "high-intensity" means to you; your rate of perceived exertion should be around eight, and you shouldn't be able to carry on a conversation. Your body's ability to swap oxygen and carbon dioxide will be reduced, and you should feel the "burn" as your body eliminates lactic acid and your muscles start to lose their ability to contract. You should be working so hard that you aren't physically able to continue this level of intensity for long.

3. After a few minutes, reduce the intensity level to something you can maintain for a longer period, but don't slow down so much that your pulse dips too low because that will cause you to completely lose the aerobic effect. This slowdown is called the active recovery period. Your body increases the exchange of oxygen and carbon dioxide to deliver nutrients to your muscles. The lactic acid burn should diminish, and your breathing rate should slow a bit. After you complete this period for a few minutes, you have accomplished one cycle.

4. Repeat this process of feeling the burn and recovering for at least thirty minutes. The high-intensity periods should be shorter than the active-recovery periods, particularly when you first start. For example, when you begin to introduce your body to interval training, walk for five minutes and then run for one minute. As you become more proficient, increase the time you spend in high-intensity periods.

Here's why high-intensity interval training is awesome:

- **It saves time.** If you normally spend an hour and a half in the gym following the "fat-burning zone" philosophy, you'll work yourself just as hard in forty-five minutes with interval training.

- **It increases metabolism.** Higher intensities stimulate your metabolism far more after the workouts than lower-intensity training. This means you continue to burn calories and fat for long periods after you're done training. This "afterburn" can burn an extra 150 to 250 calories after you stop exercising.

- **It reduces boredom.** High-intensity interval training combats boredom. It's fun, and time flies during each session because you're working in cycles of high and low intensity instead of spending a long time at any one activity. Maria likes to make a playlist of songs to match the intensity of the workout: a warm-up song, a fast-paced song, a recovery-paced song, and repeat!

- **It burns a lot of calories.** It's an aerobic workout that burns a significant number of calories.

- **It burns calories faster.** It challenges your aerobic and anaerobic systems at the same time, so you're improving your body's capacity to burn calories at a higher rate.

- **It adds new muscle.** It helps you add new muscle, which speeds up your metabolism of fat even at rest.

- **It can help you break through a weight-loss plateau.** It's effective for pushing beyond a weight-loss plateau.

Many studies have proven the value of interval training. One study followed a group of overweight women and assigned them to one of two groups. The first group worked out using high-intensity intervals, which involved two minutes of maximum effort followed by three minutes at a lower intensity. The second group worked out at a constant pace the whole time. The lengths of the workouts were varied so that both groups burned 300 calories. After the study, fitness levels in the interval group had improved by 13 percent, whereas no improvements were found in the steady-state group. The first group also continued to burn calories after the workout was finished.

HUMAN GROWTH HORMONE

Human growth hormone (HGH) is necessary for building muscle (which, in turn, increases metabolism), but it's also the fat-burning hormone. The combination of the two means that more growth hormone is great for losing weight.

Growth hormone is inversely related to insulin. If one is high, the other is low. If you eat something (especially carbohydrates) before a workout, you will be spiking your insulin level, and your growth hormone level will be low. This insulin spike is one reason it's helpful to exercise on an empty stomach or in a fasted state (see page 258 for other reasons). Short, high-intensity workouts are also awesome for stimulating growth hormone. Also, when you are lifting weights, that burn that you feel at the end means an increase in growth hormone.

CIRCUIT TRAINING: STRENGTH + CARDIO

Circuit training is a combination of strength training and cardiovascular exercise. If you're looking for a workout that provides all-over fitness benefits—from revving up your metabolism to extending your endurance—look no further than circuit training.

A circuit workout combines cardio activity like jogging with a resistance workout, with little to no rest between exercises. The absence of long rest periods makes circuit training as effective as a cardio-based high-intensity interval workout (see page 253), which raises your heart rate and boosts metabolism by building muscles. Like interval training, circuit training burns a ton of calories, not just during the workout but for hours afterward. The continued calorie-burn is called the afterburn effect. Minimizing rest time between exercises is as important as the exercises themselves. The more downtime between movements, the more your heart rate and metabolic rate decrease.

Here is a circuit-training workout that's an efficient way to burn fat:

1. Warm up for five minutes and then jog for five minutes.
    - **First rep:** Do ten push-ups and then ten sit-ups.
    - **Second rep:** Do nine push-ups and then nine sit-ups.
    - **Third rep:** Do eight push-ups and then eight sit-ups.
    - **Following reps:** Seven, six, five . . . all the way down to one rep each.

2. Jog for another five minutes.
   - **First rep:** Do ten triceps dips and then ten bicep curls.
   - **Second rep:** Do nine triceps dips and then nine bicep curls.
   - **Following reps:** Eight, seven, six . . . all the way down to one rep each.
3. Jog for another five minutes.
   - **First rep:** Do ten squats and then ten jumping jacks.
   - **Second rep:** Do nine squats and then nine jumping jacks.
   - **Following reps:** Eight, seven, six . . . all the way down to one rep each.

For a more advanced workout, repeat the whole cycle, walk to cool down, and then stretch!

YOGA

Yoga is one of the most helpful workouts for fighting stubborn fat stores. Research has found that yoga decreases levels of stress hormones and increases insulin sensitivity, which helps your body burn rather than store energy. Also, yoga can help reduce stress, bad food habits, lack of energy, and thyroid problems—all of which can be sources of weight gain.

That said, most types of yoga don't have the calorie-burning abilities of aerobic exercise. A 150-pound person will burn 150 calories in an hour of yoga compared to 311 calories in an hour of walking at three miles per hour. Yoga's best benefit when it comes to weight loss is that it puts you in touch with your body in a way nothing else can.

Yoga isn't just exercise. Yoga offers the following benefits:

- Yoga is a mind-body connection, which helps us become more in touch with our bodies and how we feel.
- Yoga creates a sense of mindfulness, which is the ability to monitor what is happening internally. You have a stronger connection to what is going on in your body.
- Yoga helps change the relationship between the mind and body, and in time, that translates into a change in eating

GOING TO BOOTCAMP

I love the circuit-training class called Bootcamp at my local gym. We rotate stations that include one strength-training activity and one cardiovascular activity, and two people share each station. For example, one station might be biceps curls for one person and explosive step-ups over an elevated step for the second person; you switch every minute or two. Once you are done with a station, you quickly do fifteen push-ups, sit-ups, or squats, and then move on to the next heart-pumping station.

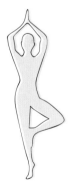

About ten years ago, I taught yoga at the Andersen Windows corporate office over the lunch hour. Just about everyone in the class was new to yoga. They mostly wanted a break from their desks and a time to relax. However, after the first class, they were surprised at how much they sweated and "felt the burn" while they were de-stressing. They were hooked. I loved hearing after each class that yoga had changed their lives in some way—they had less back pain, were making better food choices, felt happier and calmer, and more.

habits. The strong mind-body connection forged in yoga makes you more aware of what you eat and how it feels to be full, and the conscious awareness of your body translates to better appetite control. You become more aware of which foods nourish you and which make you feel lethargic.

Yoga can help you change your routine and the way you approach food or get over harmful eating patterns.

EXERCISE TIPS FOR BURNING MORE FAT

There are some tricks to exercising that can increase fat burning. Granted, these tricks won't work for everyone because we need to fit in exercise whenever we can, and some people might want to enhance performance rather than burn fat. However, if fat loss is your goal, check out these tips!

- **Exercise in the morning on an empty stomach.** If your goal is to burn fat, it's best to exercise first thing in the morning on an empty stomach. (To prevent dehydration, drink a large glass of ice water mixed with a touch of quality salt first.) Morning exercise burns 300 percent more body fat than exercising at any other time of the day because there is no glycogen (stored carbohydrates) in your liver to burn, so your body has to go directly into the fat stores to get the energy necessary to complete the activity.

THE GOAL IS A HEALTHY LIFESTYLE

Do I exercise? Yes. I run, bike, walk, lift weights, and practice yoga because I love to move. However, I did all this exercise when I was overweight, too. Nutrition was the missing key to successful weight loss.

I see exercise as a tool to help you live a healthy lifestyle. Do not push yourself by living at the gym or on a treadmill to lose more weight. A healthy lifestyle is more about what you put into your mouth than how many miles your legs can run.

- **Do cardio exercise right after weight training.** It takes twenty to thirty minutes of exercise to exhaust the glucose immediately available for fuel (unless you're working out first thing in the morning on an empty stomach—see above). It's only then that you start to burn more body fat. You deplete your glycogen stores more quickly when you do weight training exercises before cardio, which means you start burning fat sooner. Lifting weights first also means you have lots of energy to focus on correct posture, decreasing the chance of injury.

- **Change the exercise.** When you do one exercise consistently, your muscles get used to it. Workouts get easier, and those muscles don't have to work as hard, so you burn fewer calories. Frequently changing your exercise makes your muscles work harder and causes an increase in heart rate, which means an increase in calories burned.

- **Change the duration of exercise.** Changing the duration is important because you want to prevent your body from adjusting to a constant amount of activity. As soon as the body adapts to a kind of exercise, it's easier for the muscles to perform that exercise. Changes in duration also are good for performance, but it becomes tougher to reach the fat-burning zone. Extending the length of your workout can compensate.

Wear a Pedometer!

Every car has an odometer that records the miles it has traveled. Similarly, a pedometer or fitness tracker measures steps. Walking 10,000 steps a day burns 300 to 400 calories. Wearing a pedometer can enhance your motivation to increase your number of daily steps. Focus on one day at a time. Over time, you will find yourself going for an extra walk, taking extra steps from the parking lot, and expending a few more calories here and there. These small changes add up over time and lead to stable, lifelong results.

THE EXERCISE OF DAILY ACTIVITIES

There are two kinds of physical activity:

- Planned activity, such as running on a treadmill
- Unconscious movements that we perform daily, such as tapping a foot in a meeting or simply moving to get from one place to another

Both kinds of activities require fuel and affect your metabolism, which determines how your body burns fuel. Overall, activity level makes up 15 to 30 percent of your metabolism.

However, we often overestimate how much fuel we really burn during planned exercise. To put it in perspective, a runner burns about 2,500 calories during a marathon, and it takes 3,500 calories to burn one pound of fat! Plus, it can be difficult to make time for exercise; we're all so busy, it can be hard to get in three one-hour workouts a week. Here's the good news: The calories burned during unplanned activity can add up fast. Going to the grocery store and cooking dinner (versus being sedentary and ordering takeout) can burn as many calories as a boring thirty-minute run on a treadmill.

Don't misunderstand what we're saying. Exercise strengthens your heart, lungs, and muscles, which is important for overall health. Recent studies have found that exercise is more helpful in treating depression than antidepressant medications.[2] However, when it comes to weight loss, exercise is not everything.

THE DANGERS OF TOO MUCH EXERCISE

Most people do cardiovascular exercise to lose weight. Unfortunately, too much cardio stimulates cortisol, a stress hormone that tells your body to hang onto fat stores. Cortisol is released when the body is under stress. Stress from work, family life, lack of sleep, poor eating habits, and, yes, excess exercise (such as marathon training) can all stimulate cortisol.

Chronically high levels of cortisol interfere with weight loss, and they increase your risk for a variety of health issues, such as depression, sleep disturbances, and digestive issues. Also, cortisol and testosterone conflict with each other; the more aerobic work you do, the more cortisol is released and the less testosterone is available to build muscle. Plus, men suffering from lower testosterone suffer libido issues and erectile function.

Aside from cutting back on excessive, intense exercise, there's a simple way to lower cortisol: get more sleep! Some people tend to gain weight in the summer because the longer days lead to not getting enough sleep.

Stress, whether from excess cardio or other life stressors, also affects neurotransmitters such as serotonin, GABA, and dopamine. These neurotransmitters are our feel-good, antianxiety brain chemicals, and burning them out with stress and too much intense exercise can lead to depression, chronic fatigue, and sleep disorders. Also, a shortage of these neurotransmitters can cause serious thyroid conditions, such as hypothyroidism, which is known to cause weight gain, depression, and digestive dysfunction. Plus, low serotonin levels are associated with cravings for carbohydrates and binge eating.

If you are already living a life filled with stress from work, school, or family, know that exercise is another stressor. True, exercise is known to be more of a "healthy stress," but your adrenal

THE TROUBLE WITH OVERTRAINING

I love to exercise for many reasons. I enjoy my morning runs in the country because of the silence, the sights of deer, and the feeling of gratitude I get. However, it took me years to enjoy running. When I first started, even a half mile was tough for me. Now, I run every morning without difficulty, and I do it because I enjoy running, not because I am trying to lose weight.

However, eight years ago, I signed up for a marathon for weight loss, and I *gained* weight, even though I was eating the same low-carb diet and running twice a day. I was overtraining, and my high-intensity exercise routine pushed my body's stress response too far, which led to a cascade of biochemical responses that damaged my health. Pushing the body too hard can lead to higher cortisol levels, adrenal fatigue, and more hunger.

glands don't know the difference. If you have adrenal fatigue, you might want to jump to the section on yoga earlier in this chapter (see page 257). Yoga is a great low-impact exercise that can also help you de-stress.

EXERCISING IN KETOSIS

Some people are more focused on the number on the scale than on "fat" loss. The majority of "fat" in your body (over 80 percent) is collected in one form and stored in body fat cells. To get rid of it, you can use it for energy, which is a process called lipolysis. However, if you are a sugar burner—meaning that you fuel your body with carbs before you exercise—you don't initiate the production of HGH to burn fat; you primarily burn sugar. And if your body runs out and you don't keep fueling it with sugar, your body will start to break down muscle to make more sugar.

A ketogenic diet spares protein from being oxidized, which preserves muscle. Branched-chain amino acids (BCAAs) come from animal proteins and are considered essential because your body can't make them. That means you need to consume branched-chain amino acids for proper muscle building and repair (as well as replenishing red blood cells). We find it interesting that BCAA oxidation rates usually rise with exercise, which means that you need more if you are an athlete. However, keto-adapted athletes burn ketones instead of BCAAs. Critics of low-carb diets claim that the body needs insulin to grow muscles. However, in a well-designed low-carb, high-fat diet, there is less protein oxidation and double the fat oxidation, which leaves your muscles in place while all you burn is fat!

Migratory birds and whales rely on stored fat to fuel their long, strenuous journeys. Developing your fat engine will increase the amount of energy you can generate, reduce the amount of carbs you use, and stretch out the glycogen supply during long runs. When combined, you have a more stable and enduring energy supply, better endurance, and faster finish times.

Ketosis also decreases the buildup of lactate, which helps control pH and respiratory function. A myth of low-carb diets is that they put you in a state of ketoacidosis.

In *The Art and Science of Low Carb Performance,* authors Jeff S. Volek and Stephen D. Phinney state that many doctors mistake nutritional ketosis (marked by blood ketone levels of 0.5 to 5.0 millimoles per liter) for diabetic ketoacidosis, which is marked by blood ketone levels higher than 15 millimoles. They say:

> In nutritional ketosis, blood pH at rest stays normal, plus sharp drops in pH due to CO_2 and lactate buildup during exercise are restrained. By contrast, in ketoacidosis, blood pH is driven abnormally low by the 10-fold greater buildup of ketones. Suggesting these two states are similar is like equating a gentle rain with a flood because they both involve water.[3]

We know that some people reading this book believe they don't have time to exercise or don't really need to exercise. If you are one of these people, you should know that these thoughts are your brain sabotaging your efforts to improve your health. Your brain might also tell you that your healthy eating plan can wait until Monday or that one more cookie won't make a difference. We all have coping strategies to rationalize the choices we make, even though we know we are just making excuses. The trick is to realize when you are lying to yourself and not listen to that voice of negativity. Learning to ignore your negativity is a very important part of making positive changes in any area of life, including exercise. We love this statement from Carol Welch:

> Movement is medicine for changing a person's physical, emotional, and mental state.

Metabolism's third and most controllable "piece of the pie" is your activity level, which includes planned activity, such as running on a treadmill, as well as the unconscious movements that you perform daily, such as tapping your foot in a meeting. Your activity level makes up 15 to 30 percent of your metabolism.

This piece of the pie is way overappreciated. We often console our bodies with food after a hard workout. To put it in perspective, a runner burns about 2,500 calories during a marathon, and it takes 3,500 calories to burn just 1 pound of fat. The average person is busy with work and family and is lucky to get in three hour-long workouts a week. To put that in perspective, the three hours

My mom often reminds me that my grandparents always ate dessert. I remind her that they worked on a farm all day. Could you imagine their faces if they saw people running on a stationary piece of metal, staring at a television screen for an hour? Oh yeah, they also made their pies with real fats and sugar, not with Crisco and high-fructose corn syrup!

spent working out represents only 2 percent of the week. We are not trying to discourage you; we just want you to be aware that unplanned activity can add up fast. Going to the grocery store and cooking dinner can burn as many calories as running on a boring treadmill for thirty minutes!

Instead of going to the gym after work, stressing out on the way home because you don't have anything planned for dinner, and stopping at restaurant to pick up a meal, you should go to the grocery store, power shop, and make your family a healthy meal! You'll have burned the same number of calories as you would have by going to the gym, and you'll be giving your body the healthy fuel it needs to thrive.

Also, there is no need to complain that healthy eating costs too much because you just saved a ton of money by not buying frozen junk food that's been heated up at a restaurant. It's all about priorities. We don't blink an eye when we pay $20 for a restaurant pizza, but $12 for a free-range chicken is too much? This is the wrong mentality for a healthy body. The majority of our clients find that eating this way saves them money on their monthly food bill. Intermittent fasting and eating only two meals a day instead of three helps offset the cost of organic foods. Also, a dozen organic eggs typically costs about $5, and that is three meals' worth of eggs. No restaurant dish can compete with that price! Eating at home can take more time, but it costs less.

So get off the couch and increase your unplanned activity. Start wearing a pedometer, and we're sure you will surprise yourself at just how many extra steps you start taking.

If you are working out to lose weight, you must understand that weight loss is all about hormone manipulation and the health of your mitochondria. The best way to burn fat is to perform aerobic exercise first thing in the morning on an empty stomach after drinking a large glass of water with a bit of quality salt, to avoid dehydration.

Focus on your diet first, and add small movements throughout the day. As you lose weight and your energy increases, start some of the strength training and other activities outlined in this chapter. Think of these workouts as a long-term investment in your health. Working out and building a strong body now will ensure that you have a more active and healthy lifestyle as you age.

EXERCISE HELPS BREAK BAD HABITS

Habits are hard to break. Instead of just stopping a bad habit, we like to help people form new, healthier habits. Only cutting out the bad habit can set you up for failure. However, replacing those bad habits with better habits creates success! This is where exercise can be an effective tool. Instead of sitting around and eating a bedtime snack, we suggest a bedtime yoga routine to help calm your mind and body. Maria grew up with a bedtime snack routine, and it was the hardest habit for her to break. Practicing a bedtime yoga routine has really helped her, and many of our clients, replace that unhealthy snack with a mind- and body-enhancing routine.

chapter 11

Meal Plans and Pantry List

Following a ketogenic diet can be really easy once you know which foods you can eat and stay in ketosis. This chapter will help you give your refrigerator, freezer, and pantry a makeover. Here, we provide some shopping tips, along with a no-bake seven-day meal plan and even a no-bake nut-free, dairy-free seven-day meal plan, with a grocery list for each plan.

STOCKING YOUR REFRIGERATOR, FREEZER, AND PANTRY

The key to any healthy diet is eating real, whole foods. In the ketogenic lifestyle, you'll want to seek out certain ingredients and avoid others.

Purchasing Keto-Friendly Ingredients

You can purchase keto-friendly pantry products on our website, MariaMindBodyHealth.com/store. They're also available at most grocery stores.

To save money, we recommend buying ingredients in bulk—including perishables like meat and fresh veggies. They can be frozen (a chest freezer is a great investment!) and thawed when you are ready to use them.

Remember, choosing the best-quality organic foods is always optimal.

PROTEINS

It's always best to choose grass-fed, organic, and humanely raised meat and wild-caught seafood. These options not only offer more nutrients, but also haven't been exposed to added hormones, antibiotics, or other potential toxins.

For help in choosing sustainably sourced seafood, check out the Monterey Bay Aquarium Seafood Watch app and website, seafoodwatch.org.

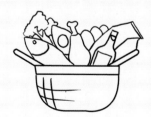

BEEF	FISH	SEAFOOD/SHELLFISH	POULTRY	EGGS
• Ground beef	• Ahi	• Clams	• Chicken	• Chicken eggs
• Steak	• Catfish	• Crab	• Duck	• Duck eggs
BUFFALO	• Halibut	• Lobster	• Game hen	• Goose eggs
	• Herring	• Mussels	• Goose	• Ostrich eggs
GOAT	• Mackerel	• Oysters	• Ostrich	• Quail eggs
LAMB	• Mahi mahi	• Prawns	• Partridge	
PORK	• Salmon	• Scallops	• Pheasant	
	• Sardines	• Shrimp	• Quail	
WILD MEATS	• Snapper	• Snails	• Squab	
• Bear	• Swordfish		• Turkey	
• Boar	• Trout			
• Elk	• Tuna			
• Rabbit	• Walleye			
• Venison	• White fish (such as cod)			

TIP

A chest freezer is great for keeping food fresh for months. It also enables you to store larger quantities when you find discounted prices. We highly recommend that you get one! We also recommend ButcherBox and Sizzlefish, both of which will deliver quality proteins to your door.

Also, many people see great benefits from including collagen in their diet. It helps tighten loose skin, reverse the aging of skin, promote hair growth, and improve joint health, and it is a great prebiotic for keeping your gut flora healthy. We like the Further Foods brand because it is grass-fed and has no flavor, so it can be added to any food (or even water).

DAIRY

Dairy can be a part of a well-formulated ketogenic diet, but our clients do see better results when they eliminate dairy for the first thirty days or so. Doing so gives the gut a chance to heal from any irritation or inflammation that past dairy consumption may have caused. Eliminating dairy (as well as nuts) can also be helpful for breaking through a weight-loss stall.

You can test yourself for dairy tolerance after you have eliminated it for a month or so. Weigh yourself in the morning, consume a small amount of dairy later that day, and then weigh yourself again the next morning. If you gained weight (that is, retained water), then you are still sensitive to dairy and should continue to avoid it for at least another month.

If you want to try reintroducing dairy to your diet after a month or more of being dairy-free, choose just one item and see how your body responds to it over two or three days. If you don't have any reaction, chances are you're not dairy sensitive.

It is always best to purchase grass-fed and organic dairy products from humanely raised animals if you can. Here is a list of keto-approved dairy products:

- Butter
- Ghee*
- Crème fraîche
- Heavy cream
- Sour cream
- Cream cheese
- Mascarpone cheese
- Cheeses (Burrata, Brie, blue cheese, cheddar, feta, Gouda, Halloumi, Havarti, Manchego, mozzarella, Monterey Jack, Provolone, Roquefort, cheese curds, queso fresco)
- Hard cheeses (Asiago, Parmesan, aged Gouda, Romano, aged cheddar, fontina)

Ghee can be a good fat to use even if you are dairy sensitive because the milk proteins have been removed.

Consume these dairy products in moderation, as their carbs can add up quickly:

- Cottage cheese
- Ricotta cheese

Avoid these dairy products, which have too many carbs:

- Buttermilk
- Condensed or evaporated milk
- Cow's milk
- Whey protein powder*
- Yogurt

Whey protein can raise blood sugar much more than other proteins when it is isolated into a protein powder. For this reason, we recommend that you opt for other types of protein powder, such as egg white protein or plant protein.

FATS

On a keto diet, you need lots of healthy fat to burn as fuel. But as important as it is to seek out healthy fats, it's just as critical to avoid unhealthy fats.

Healthy Fats

Fats with high amounts of saturated fatty acids (SFAs)—such as MCT oil, coconut oil, tallow, and lard—are best; they are stable and anti-inflammatory, are less likely to oxidize, and have many other important health benefits. Look for grass-fed and organic sources. Try to avoid polyunsaturated fatty acids (PUFAs), which are prone to oxidation and therefore are less healthy. (We talk more about unhealthy fats on page 272.)

Below is a list of the best oils and fats to use, with their SFA and PUFA contents. When choosing a fat, make sure to take into account whether you need it for a hot or a cold use.

FAT	SFA	PUFA	NOTES
Almond oil	8.2%	17%	• Has a mild, neutral flavor • Works great for sweet dishes and Thai dishes • Use in nonheat applications, such as salad dressings • Can be used on the skin
Avocado oil	11%	10%	• Has a mild, neutral flavor • Works great for savory and sweet dishes, as well as Thai dishes • Can be heated
Beef tallow	49.8%	3.1%	• Has a mild beef flavor • Works great for savory dishes • Can be heated
Cocoa butter	60%	3%	• Has a mild coconut flavor • Works great for sweet and savory cooking • Can be heated
Coconut oil	92%	1.9%	• Has a strong coconut flavor • Works great for sweet dishes and Thai dishes • Can be heated • Can be used on the skin

FAT	SFA	PUFA	NOTES
Duck fat	25%	13%	• Has a rich duck flavor • Works great for frying savory foods • Can be heated
Extra-virgin olive oil*	14%	9.9%	• Has a strong olive flavor • Works great for Italian salad dressings • Use in nonheat applications, such as salad dressings
Hazelnut oil	10%	14%	• Has a mild hazelnut flavor • Works great for sweet dishes and Thai dishes • Use in nonheat applications, such as salad dressings
High oleic sunflower oil	8%	9%	• Has a mild sunflower seed flavor • Works great for sweet dishes and Thai dishes • Use in nonheat applications, such as salad dressings
Lard	41%	12%	• Has a mild flavor • Works great for frying sweet or savory foods • Can be heated
Macadamia nut oil	15%	10%	• Has a mild nutty flavor • Works great for salad dressings • Use in nonheat applications, such as salad dressings
MCT oil**	97%	less than 1%	• Has a neutral flavor • Works in savory dishes and baked goods • Can be heated to low or moderate heat (no higher than 320°F)
Palm kernel oil***	82%	2%	• Has a neutral flavor • Works great for baking • Can be heated

*Extra-virgin olive oil is great for cold applications, such as salad dressings, but do not use it for cooking; heat causes the oil to oxidize, which is harmful to your health.

**MCT oil can be found at most health-food stores, but if you have trouble finding it, you can use avocado oil, macadamia nut oil, or extra-virgin olive oil instead, keeping in mind that avocado oil is the most neutral-flavored of the three.

***Be sure to purchase sustainably sourced and processed palm kernel oil. There are ecological concerns associated with some palm oils.

If you're not dairy sensitive, the following are great healthy, keto-friendly dairy fats to add to your diet:

FAT	SFA	PUFA
Butter	50%	3.4%
Ghee*	48%	4%
Heavy cream	62%	4%
Cream cheese	56%	4%
Cheese	64%	3%
Sour cream	58%	4%
Crème fraîche	64%	3%

Unhealthy Fats

Two kinds of fats should be avoided on a ketogenic diet: trans fats and polyunsaturated fatty acids (PUFAs).

Trans fats are the most inflammatory fats; in fact, they are among the worst substances for our health that we can consume. Many studies have shown that eating foods containing trans fats increases the risk of heart disease and cancer.

Here is a list of trans fats to avoid at all costs:

- Hydrogenated or partially hydrogenated oils (check ingredient labels)
- Margarine
- Vegetable shortening

PUFAs should also be limited, as they are prone to oxidation. Many cooking oils are high in PUFAs. Below is a list of the most common ones.

FAT	PUFA
Grapeseed oil	70.6%
Sunflower oil	68%
Flax oil	66%
Safflower oil	65%
Soybean oil	58%
Corn oil	54.6%
Walnut oil	53.9%
Cottonseed oil	52.4%
Vegetable oil	51.4%
Sesame oil	42%
Peanut oil	33.4%
Canola oil	19%

BEVERAGES

It probably goes without saying that soda and fruit juice should be avoided on a keto diet—they're full of sugars that will raise your blood sugar and kick you out of ketosis. But that doesn't mean you're limited to just water! The following are liquids that you can consume:

- Unsweetened almond milk
- Unsweetened cashew milk
- Unsweetened coconut milk
- Unsweetened hemp milk
- Green tea*
- Herbal tea*
- Organic caffè Americano (espresso with water)*
- Mineral water
- Water (reverse osmosis is best)
- Zevia soda

Consume caffeine in moderation. If weight loss is a goal, consider removing all caffeine.

> TIP
> We love Everly water enhancers, which add flavor to plain water.

NUTS AND SEEDS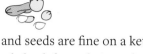

Moderate amounts of nuts and seeds are fine on a ketogenic diet, but they can hold some people back from their goals. If weight loss is a goal for you, we recommend removing nuts and seeds to improve your results.

Here is a list of keto-friendly nuts and seeds that you can enjoy when you are closer to your goal weight:

NUT/SEED TYPE	CARB COUNT PER 1-OUNCE SERVING
Pili nuts	1g
Brazil nuts	3g
Sesame seeds	3g
Pecans	4g
Macadamia nuts	4g
Pumpkin seeds	4g
Walnuts	4g
Hazelnuts	5g
Pine nuts	5g
Almonds	6g
Sunflower seeds	6g

Butters made from these nuts and seeds are good options as well. Just look for products made with only nuts, salt, and any of the natural sweeteners listed in the sweetener section.

Some nuts are very high in carbs and should be avoided. Here is a list of the nuts we do not recommend:

- Cashews (9 grams of carbs per 1-ounce serving)
- Pistachios (8 grams of carbs per 1-ounce serving)
- Chestnuts (22 grams of carbs per 1-ounce serving)

Also, avoid flax seeds, flax meal, and chia seeds (along with all soy products), as they are high in phytoestrogens that can mess up hormone balance and raise bad estrogen levels.

VEGETABLES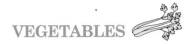

Fresh vegetables are packed with nutrients and are an important part of a keto lifestyle, but to make sure that you stay in ketosis, it's important to choose nonstarchy vegetables, which are lower in carbs. The following are some of the nonstarchy vegetables that we use most:

- Arugula
- Asparagus
- Bok choy
- Broccoli
- Cabbage
- Cauliflower
- Celery
- Collard greens
- Endive
- Garlic
- Kale
- Kelp

- Lettuce: red leaf, Boston, romaine, radicchio
- Mushrooms
- Onions: green, yellow, white, red
- Peppers: bell peppers, jalapeños, chiles
- Radishes
- Seaweed
- Spinach
- Swiss chard
- Watercress

Limit these veggies, as carbs can add up quickly:

- Brussels sprouts
- Green beans
- Pumpkin

Avoid these veggies:

- Carrots
- Corn
- Green peas
- Leeks
- Parsnips

- Potatoes
- Squash
- Sweet potatoes
- Yams
- Yuca

HERBS AND SPICES

Spices and fresh herbs are the most nutritious plants you can consume. For example, everyone thinks spinach is an amazingly nutritious food, but fresh oregano has eight times its amount of antioxidants! Sure, we don't eat a cup of oregano, but it does go to show that a little bit of an herb provides a huge benefit.

- Anise
- Annatto
- Basil
- Bay leaf
- Black pepper
- Caraway
- Cardamom
- Cayenne pepper
- Celery seed
- Chervil
- Chili pepper
- Chives
- Cilantro
- Cinnamon

- Cloves
- Coriander
- Cumin
- Curry
- Dill
- Fenugreek
- Galangal
- Garlic
- Ginger
- Lemongrass
- Licorice
- Mace
- Marjoram
- Mint

- Mustard seeds
- Oregano
- Paprika
- Parsley
- Peppermint
- Rosemary
- Saffron
- Sage
- Spearmint
- Star anise
- Tarragon
- Thyme
- Turmeric
- Vanilla beans

FRUIT

We tend to think of fruit as a health food, but in reality, most fruits are full of carbs and sugar. In fact, studies prove that the produce we consume today is lower in nutrients and much higher in sugar than it was in Paleolithic times. In general, high-sugar fruits like grapes, bananas, and mangoes should be avoided during your keto cleanse.

But that doesn't mean you have to avoid all fruits! Maria once made a keto fruit salad filled with cucumbers, olives, eggplant, and capers, all covered in a Greek vinaigrette. So, yes, fruits are certainly allowed. Just seek out those that are low in sugar:

- Avocados
- Cucumbers
- Eggplants

- Lemons
- Limes
- Olives

- Seasonal wild berries (consume in moderation and for maintenance, not weight loss)
- Tomatoes (consume in moderation for weight loss)
- Zucchini

BAKING PRODUCTS

See pages 279 to 282 for recommended sweeteners.

- Baking soda
- Blanched almond flour
- Cocoa butter
- Coconut flour
- Egg white protein powder (check carbs and added ingredients—we recommend Jay Robb brand)
- Extracts and essential oils, including pure vanilla extract, for flavoring

- Pecan meal
- Unsweetened baking chocolate
- Unsweetened cocoa powder
- Whey protein powder (check carbs and added ingredients; do not use if dairy sensitive)
- Xanthan gum/guar gum

SAUCES AND FLAVOR ENHANCERS

- Apple cider vinegar
- Coconut aminos
- Coconut vinegar
- Fish sauce
- Organic tamari

KETO EGG REPLACER

The only keto egg replacer that we recommend is gelatin. Simply dissolve 1 tablespoon of grass-fed gelatin into 1 tablespoon of room-temperature or cold water. Then add 2 tablespoons of hot water and stir until dissolved and frothy. This replaces one egg. Chia and flax seeds are not recommended because of their estrogenic properties as well as their high carb counts.

CANNED, JARRED, AND PACKAGED FOODS

It is always better to buy fresh ingredients, but here are some keto-friendly foods that are also great in cans, jars, or packages:

- Adapt bars
- Banana peppers
- Beef sticks like EPIC bars (made from grass-fed meat—check flavors for added sugars)
- Boxed beef and chicken broth
- Canned anchovies
- Canned coconut milk
- Canned oysters
- Canned salmon
- Canned sardines
- Canned tuna
- Capers
- Fat Snax cookies
- Fermented pickles*
- Fermented sauerkraut*
- Keto Kookies
- Marinara sauce (watch out for vegetable oils and added sugars)**

- Mikey's English Muffins
- Nori wraps
- Olives (choose jarred over canned)
- Paleo mayonnaise (watch out for vegetable oils)
- Paleo salad dressings like ranch or Caesar (watch out for vegetable oils and added sugars)
- Pickled eggs
- Pickled herring
- Pizza sauce (watch out for vegetable oils and added sugar)
- Pure Wraps
- Sardines
- Tomato paste**
- Tomato sauce**
- Xanthan gum and guar gum (thickeners)

*Not only is fermenting a great way to preserve food, but it also creates beneficial gut bacteria and helpful digestive enzymes. Fermented sauerkraut is particularly rich in B vitamins.

**Buy jarred, not canned, tomato products whenever possible. The lining of cans contains BPA, a chemical that's associated with several health problems and may affect children's development, and tomatoes' high acidity can cause more BPA to leach into the food.

NATURAL SWEETENERS

In recipes, we always use natural sweeteners. Just as sugarcane and honey are found in nature, so are erythritol and the stevia herb. However, we prefer not to use sweeteners such as honey, maple syrup, and agave because even though they're natural, they raise blood sugar, which not only causes inflammation but will also take you out of ketosis. A list of where common sweeteners fall on the glycemic index is below.

GLYCEMIC INDEX OF SWEETENERS	
Swerve	0
Erythritol	0
Monk fruit	0
Yacón syrup	1
Xylitol	7
Agave	13
Maple syrup	54
Honey	62
Table sugar	68
Splenda	80
HFCS	87

Fructose is particularly problematic. More than glucose, it promotes a chemical reaction called glycation, which results in advanced glycation end-products (AGEs). AGEs form a sort of crust around cells that has been linked with a wide range of diseases, from diabetes and heart disease to asthma, polycystic ovary syndrome, and Alzheimer's disease. Fructose also contributes to nonalcoholic fatty liver disease. For these reasons, we avoid sweeteners that are high in fructose: table sugar, high-fructose corn syrup, honey, agave, and maple syrup.

But sugar is hidden in many products under many names. Be a detective and read those labels! Watch out for these sneaky sugars:

brown sugar, corn syrup, corn syrup solids, dextrose, fructose, fruit juice concentrate, glucose, honey, invert sugar, lactose, malt syrup, molasses, raw sugar, sucrose, maple syrup, brown rice syrup, agave nectar, beet sugar, cane crystals, corn sweetener, dehydrated cane juice, dextrin, high-fructose corn syrup (HFCS), maltose (anything ending in "-ose" is a sugar!), palm sugar, saccharose, sorghum or sorghum syrup, syrup, treacle, turbinado sugar, xylose

We also do not recommend artificial sweeteners, as they can affect thyroid function (sucralose) and cause other issues. They also put a load on the liver and can hold back your results. Avoid all artificial sweeteners, including sucralose, aspartame, acesulfame potassium, neotame, saccharin, and advantame.

The following is a list of the natural sweeteners that we do recommend, all of which have little effect on blood sugar. We'll talk in more detail about each type of sweetener below.

- Allulose
- Blended sweeteners (Swerve, Lakanto, Sukrin)
- Erythritol
- Monk fruit
- Stevia, liquid or powdered (without additives)
- Stevia glycerite (a thick liquid form of stevia)
- Xylitol
- Yacón syrup (in small amounts, as it does contain some fructose)

Allulose

Allulose is a new rare sugar that occurs naturally in some plants but has recently been produced in volume as a sweetener. It tastes like sugar, bakes like sugar, and has an aftertaste just like sugar. It also doesn't get hard in the freezer like erythritol does, so it is great for making ice cream. Most allulose is excreted in the urine, but some is fermented in the bowel, which can cause gas, bloating, and other symptoms. Use it in moderation.

Blended Sweeteners

Many brands combine two or more natural sweeteners to get a more balanced flavor. Here are a couple of good blended sweeteners:

- **Swerve** is a zero-calorie sweetener that combines erythritol (opposite) and oligosaccharides, which are prebiotic fibers found in starchy root vegetables. Swerve is nonglycemic and therefore does not affect blood sugar. It also measures cup for cup just like table sugar. It has a bit of a cooling effect in the aftertaste.

- **Lakanto** blends erythritol and monk fruit and has a balanced aftertaste.

Erythritol

Despite its chemical-sounding name, erythritol is not an artificial sweetener. It's a sugar alcohol that is found naturally in some fruits and fermented foods. Erythritol is a calorie-free sweetener that doesn't raise blood sugar or insulin, and because it's almost completely absorbed before it reaches the colon, it doesn't cause as much digestive upset as other sugar alcohols can.

Erythritol is generally available in granulated form, though sometimes you can find it powdered. If you purchase granulated erythritol, we recommend grinding it to a powder before using. In its granulated form, erythritol doesn't dissolve well and can give dishes a grainy texture.

Monk Fruit

Also known as lo han kuo, monk fruit is cultivated in the mountains of southern China. Similar to stevia, it's 300 times sweeter than sugar, but unlike stevia, it doesn't have a bitter aftertaste. Monk fruit comes in pure liquid form and in powdered form.

Since it is so much sweeter than sugar, the powdered form of monk fruit is typically bulked up with another sweetener so that it measures cup for cup like sugar. Check the ingredients for things like maltodextrin and only buy brands that use keto-friendly sweeteners, such as erythritol.

Stevia

Stevia is available as a powder or a liquid. Because stevia is so concentrated, many companies add bulking agents like maltodextrin to powdered stevia so that it's easier to bake with. Stay away from those products. Table sugar has a glycemic index of

52, whereas maltodextrin has a glycemic index of 110!

Look for products that contain just stevia or stevia combined with another natural and keto-friendly sweetener.

Stevia Glycerite

Stevia glycerite is a thick liquid form of stevia that is similar in consistency to honey. Do not confuse it with liquid stevia, which is much more concentrated. Stevia glycerite is about twice as sweet as sugar, making it a bit less sweet than pure liquid or powdered stevia. We prefer to use stevia glycerite because, unlike the powdered or liquid forms of stevia, it has no bitter aftertaste.

Stevia glycerite is great for cooking because it maintains flavor that many other sweeteners lose when heated. However, it doesn't caramelize or create bulk, so most baking recipes call for combining it with another sweetener.

Xylitol

Xylitol is a naturally occurring low-calorie sweetener found in fruits and vegetables. It has a minimal effect on blood sugar and insulin. While it's not as low on the glycemic index as erythritol, erythritol doesn't work well for low-carb hard candies (it doesn't melt properly), so we use xylitol instead.

Xylitol has been known to kick some people out of ketosis, so if you're using it for baking or cooking, monitor your ketones closely and stop using it if you find that you're no longer in ketosis.

Yacón Syrup

Yacón syrup is a thick syrup that is pressed from the yacón root and tastes a bit like molasses. It has been consumed for centuries in Peru.

We use yacón syrup sparingly, both because it is very expensive and because it has some fructose in it. A small jar lasts us four to six months. We use a tablespoon here and there to improve the texture and flavor of sauces; it's ideal for giving sweet-and-sour sauce that perfect mouthfeel or giving BBQ sauce a hint of molasses. Using these small amounts keeps the sugar content to 1 gram or so per serving.

NO-COOK 7-DAY MEAL PLAN

MEAL PLAN

	BREAKFAST	SNACK	DINNER	Nutrition Facts Per Serving
DAY 1	3 hard-boiled eggs, 4 ounces boneless salmon	1 cup pork rinds, ½ cup salsa	4 ounces turkey, 2 medium lettuce leaves, ¼ cup mayonnaise, ½ cup grated sharp cheddar cheese	Calories 1224 Fat 89g Carbs 6g Protein 97g
DAY 2	8 dill pickles, 2⅓ tbsp ranch dressing, 3 ounces ham	2 (1-ounce) beef sticks	1 cup drained tuna (solid or chunks), 2 tbsp mayonnaise, 1 stalk celery, 1 hard-boiled egg, 3 medium lettuce leaves	Calories 1036 Fat 76g Carbs 3g Protein 79g
DAY 3	½ avocado, 3 ounces turkey	¼ cup pili nuts	6 ounces cooked chicken breast, 2 cups romaine lettuce, ¼ cup grated sharp cheddar cheese, ¼ cup + 2 tsp ranch dressing, ¼ medium tomato (2⅗ inches in diameter)	Calories 1178 Fat 92g Carbs 13g Protein 75g
DAY 4	Egg salad, 2 medium lettuce leaves, ¼ cup guacamole	1 (3¾-ounce) can drained sardines	6 ounces roast beef, 1 cup onion, ¼ medium (2⅗ inches in diameter) tomato, 3 medium lettuce leaves, 2 tbsp mayonnaise	Calories 1144 Fat 79g Carbs 25g Protein 75g
DAY 5	3 hard-boiled eggs, 3 ounces ham	1 cup black olives	6 ounces boneless smoked salmon, 4 medium lettuce leaves, ¼ cup + 2 tsp ranch dressing, ¼ cup onion, ½ bell pepper	Calories 1098 Fat 87g Carbs 13g Protein 70g
DAY 6	½ avocado, 3 ounces turkey	2 (1-ounce) beef sticks, 1 cup black olives	1 cup drained tuna (solid or chunks), 2 tbsp mayonnaise, 1 stalk celery, 1 hard-boiled egg, 3 medium lettuce leaves	Calories 1063 Fat 74g Carbs 14g Protein 88g
DAY 7	3 hard-boiled eggs, 4 ounces boneless smoked salmon	¼ cup pili nuts	6 ounces cubed ham, ¼ cup grated sharp cheddar cheese, 6 medium lettuce leaves, ¼ cup onion, ¼ cup + 2 tsp ranch dressing	Calories 1124 Fat 89g Carbs 11g Protein 80g

GROCERY LIST

Use this grocery list to shop for the No-Cook 7-Day Meal Plan. The Quantity column lists the amount you need to purchase and shows the amount needed for the recipes—if only a portion is used—in parentheses.

INGREDIENT	QUANTITY
Baking Products	
Pili nuts	¼ cup
Canned/Jarred Items	
Dill pickles	1 jar (8 pickles)
Olives, black	2 cups
Tuna, solid or chunks	2 cups
Condiments	
Dijon mustard (for egg salad)	2 tablespoons
Mayonnaise	1 jar (19 tablespoons)
Ranch dressing	1 jar (17½ tablespoons)
Salsa	½ cup
Eggs and Dairy	
Eggs	19 large (including 11 hard-boiled)
Sharp cheddar cheese	1 cup shredded
Prepackaged Items	
Beef sticks (check for added sugar; we like the Paleo Valley brand)	3 (1 ounce each)
Guacamole	1 package (¼ cup)
Pork rinds	1 bag

INGREDIENT	QUANTITY
Produce	
Avocado	1 whole
Bell pepper	½ medium
Celery	2 stalks
Fresh dill (for egg salad)	1 tablespoon
Leaf lettuce	1 large head
Onion	1 medium (1½ cups)
Romaine lettuce	1 large head
Tomato	½ medium
Proteins	
Cubed ham	6 ounces
Deli chicken breast	6 ounces
Deli ham	9 ounces
Deli turkey breast	11 ounces
Sardines	1 (3¾-ounce) can
Smoked salmon (boneless)	14 ounces

NO-COOK 7-DAY DAIRY- AND NUT-FREE MEAL PLAN

MEAL PLAN

	BREAKFAST	SNACK	DINNER	Nutrition Facts Per Serving
DAY 1	3 hard-boiled eggs, 4 ounces boneless smoked salmon	1 cup pork rinds, ½ cup salsa	4 ounces turkey, 2 medium lettuce leaves, ¼ cup mayonnaise, ½ cup diced tomatoes	Calories 1028 Fat 71g Carbs 8g Protein 84g
DAY 2	8 dill pickles, 2½ tablespoons dairy-free ranch dressing 3 ounces ham	2 (1-ounce) beef sticks	1 cup drained tuna (solid or chunks), 3 tbsp mayonnaise, 1 stalk celery, 1 hard-boiled egg, 3 medium lettuce leaves	Calories 1104 Fat 84g Carbs 3g Protein 79g
DAY 3	½ avocado, 3 ounces turkey	1 cup black olives	6 ounces cooked chicken breast, 2 cups romaine lettuce, ½ cup diced tomatoes, 1 tablespoon dairy-free ranch dressing	Calories 1062 Fat 75g Carbs 19g Protein 74g
DAY 4	Egg salad with dairy-free ranch dressing, 2 medium lettuce leaves, ¼ cup guacamole	1 (3¾-ounce) can sardines, drained	6 ounces roast beef, 1 cup onion, ¼ medium tomato (2⅗ inches in diameter), 2 medium lettuce leaves, 2 tbsp mayonnaise	Calories 1163 Fat 82g Carbs 25g Protein 75g
DAY 5	3 hard-boiled eggs, 3 ounces ham	1 (3¾-ounce) can smoked oysters	6 ounces boneless smoked salmon, 4 medium lettuce leaves 5 tablespoons dairy-free ranch dressing, 2 (⅛-inch-thick) slices onion, ½ bell pepper	Calories 1143 Fat 79g Carbs 10g Protein 91g
DAY 6	½ avocado, 3 ounces turkey	2 (1-ounce) beef sticks, 1 cup black olives	1 cup drained tuna (solid or chunks), 3 tbsp mayonnaise, 1 stalk celery, 1 hard-boiled egg, 3 medium lettuce leaves	Calories 1173 Fat 89g Carbs 17g Protein 90g
DAY 7	3 hard-boiled eggs, 4 ounces boneless smoked salmon	1 cup pork rinds, ½ cup salsa	6 ounces cubed ham, 6 medium lettuce leaves, ½ cup onion, 3 servings dairy-free ranch dressing	Calories 1094 Fat 74g Carbs 17g Protein 90g

GROCERY LIST

Use this grocery list to shop for the 7-Day No-Cook Dairy- and Nut-Free Meal Plan. The Quantity column lists the amount you need to purchase and shows the amount needed for the recipes—if only a portion is used—in parentheses.

INGREDIENT	QUANTITY
Canned/Jarred/Boxed Items	
Dill pickles	1 jar (8 pickles)
Mayonnaise	1 jar (¾ cup)
Olives, black	2 cups
Salsa	1 jar (1 cup)
Tuna, solid or chunks	2 cups
Condiments	
Dairy-free ranch dressing (we like the Primal Kitchen brand)	1½ cups
Dijon mustard (for egg salad)	2 tablespoons
Eggs	
Eggs	19 large (including 11 hard-boiled)
Produce	
Avocado	1
Bell pepper	1 (2 slices)
Celery	2 stalks
Fresh dill (for egg salad)	1 tablespoon
Leaf lettuce	1 medium head (21 leaves)
Onion	1 medium (2 slices)
Romaine lettuce	1 head (2 cups)
Tomato	1 large (1 cup)

INGREDIENT	QUANTITY
Proteins	
Cubed ham	6 ounces
Deli chicken breast	6 ounces
Deli ham	9 ounces
Deli roast beef	6 ounces
Deli turkey breast	12 ounces
Sardines	1 can (3¾ ounces)
Smoked oysters	1 can (3¾ ounces)
Smoked salmon (boneless)	14 ounces
Prepackaged Items	
Beef sticks (check for added sugar; we like the Paleo Valley brand)	3 (1 ounce each)
Guacamole (premade)	2 tablespoons
Pork rinds	1 bag

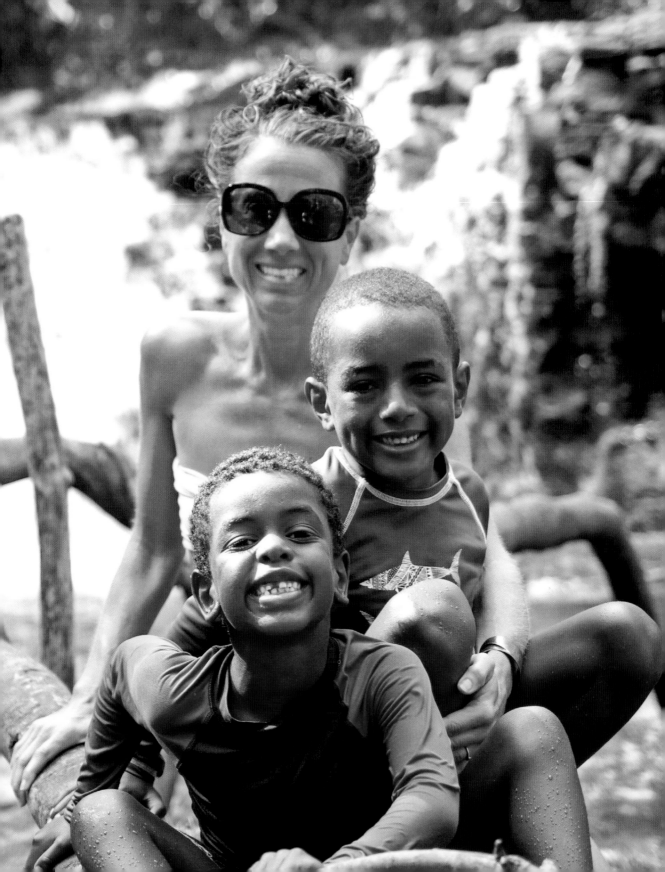

chapter 12

A Checklist for Accelerated Healing

Maria always tries to pack as many recipes into her cookbooks as she can, and sometimes that means including a bonus chapter with additional recipes. We wanted to do something similar in this book, only this time, we are adding a chapter with more steps you can take to accelerate healing and promote mitochondrial health.

COLD THERAPY AND ACTIVATING BROWN FAT

Are you always cold? Do you have a weak immune system and get sick often? Well, when was the last time you spent time in an environment that wasn't a comfortable 72°F? In our modern society, we never get to utilize our micro-muscles that are stimulated by cold temperatures.

What if we told you that to boost your immune system and enhance your sympathetic nervous system, you should push yourself into uncomfortably cold situations? It works. Even after short sessions of cold therapy, people experience remarkable increases in immune function and circulation.

Studies have shown that the blood values of people who practice cold therapy have remarkably fewer inflammatory proteins than those who live at a constantly comfortable temperature. Cold therapy conveys remarkable benefits to the immune system.

A man named Wim Hof goes by the moniker "The Iceman." When Hof exposes his body to ice, his inflammatory proteins drop to almost zero, and after only six days of exposure to ice, his white blood cells produce lower levels of cytokines (inflammatory proteins). High levels of these inflammatory proteins are directly related to increased rates of Crohn's disease, arthritis, and other autoimmune disorders.

You don't have to take cold therapy to the same extremes that The Iceman endures. He has trained his body to withstand ice-cold situations for longer than eighty minutes without risking hypothermia, which occurs when the body's temperature dips below 35°F. Hof can keep his body surface temperature at 37°F. His metabolism increases by 300 percent during his exposure to ice, which increases his body temperature so he maintains that surface

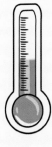

temperature of 37°F longer than he should be able to. Because of his large amount of brown fat (defined later in this section) and his years of training, Hof doesn't even shiver when he puts his body into such extremely cold situations.

We are not recommending that you start at such a level as Hof and immerse your body in ice for long periods. Something as simple as taking a cold shower (or turning the shower to cold at the end and keeping it there for as long as you can) has significant benefits. This practice alone has been proven to increase white blood cell count to help combat disease. A cold shower also helps improve circulation. Just try it!

After a cold shower, you will notice how much warmer you feel throughout the day. As another benefit, your immune system gets a huge boost. Cold therapy helps alleviate autoimmune disorders such as rheumatoid arthritis, which is caused by an overactive immune system that causes irregularities in how your body reacts and starts to attack even its own cells. Rheumatoid arthritis also causes extreme joint pain. Cold therapy helps such conditions by limiting the antibodies your immune system is producing, which in turn reduces the inflammation of the joints.

Cold therapy also offers tremendous benefits for the heart and lungs. It makes sense: When your body temperature is lower, your heart needs to pump less frequently. As we write this on a hot summer day, we're watching our dog, Ohana. She is lying here panting as if she has just chased a rabbit. When you're cold, your heart pumps less often, yet it still gets blood to all the parts of your body. Exposing yourself to the cold trains the micro-muscles within your blood vessels to work more efficiently.

Cold shrinks the mitochondria, which makes them more efficient. Cold therapy also helps with muscle repair and recovery. This is why you see football players getting ice baths after games. So give cold therapy a try. Start slow and work your way up to longer cold exposure.

There are two types of fat in the body:

- **White adipose tissue (WAT)** is what we normally refer to as body fat. We want to burn white fat.
- **Brown adipose tissue (BAT)** is composed of iron-containing mitochondria, which is best known for creating ATP (energy). More mitochondria equal more energy! BAT helps you use

excess calories for heat. Newborn babies have significant amounts of brown fat, yet overweight people have little to none. Brown fat can be activated in the presence of cold, and in the process, fatty acids are released to provide the body with the heat it needs. If you use the techniques outlined in this book, you can use BAT to your advantage, which means excess calories are not stored as WAT (which ends up as undesirable belly fat). Cold stimulates BAT to burn excess fat and glucose for energy. Brown fat is beneficial because it helps burn calories and burns unhealthy WAT.

Here are some techniques you can use to activate brown fat:

- Use ice packs on your back or neck for thirty to sixty minutes while relaxing at night, when your insulin levels are higher and you are more sensitive to insulin.

- Soak your feet in cold water at night or when you first wake up in the morning, which will stimulate your body to produce heat during the day.

- Suck on ice cubes throughout the day.

- Enjoy a snow cone with flavored stevia drops (root beer, for example) for dessert.

- Take a very cold shower upon waking or, at the end of your shower, turn the water to cold for as long as you can handle it. Try to increase your time spent under cold water a little bit each day.

- Lower the temperature in your home by 5°F.

And here are some ways to implement cold therapy:

- **Drink ice-cold water in the morning.** Ice water shrinks the mitochondria, which makes them more efficient and helps them function better.

- **Run in the cold.** Being cold is important to cellular health because it shrinks the size of the mitochondria.

- **Use cold therapy about an hour before bed.** It helps cool your body for a nice, long sleep!

DITCHING COFFEE

There was a time when I loved coffee. Heck, I worked at one coffee shop in high school and at a different one in college! However, I eventually learned about the connection between caffeine, the adrenals, hormones, and insulin. So I switched to decaf Americano, chocolate safari tea, green tea, and ice water. I also suck on ice.

HOW I PRACTICE COLD THERAPY

I start by putting my feet in a large bucket that goes as high as my knees. I fill it with ice-cold water from the hose outside, which slowly gets me used to the cold temperature. I used to try to take an ice-cold shower, but I find that starting with my feet is easier to do. Once my feet and legs are submerged in the ice water, I spray my arms, head, and back with the ice-cold water.

MORE WAYS TO HELP YOUR MITOCHONDRIA

Our bodies are complex systems with many inputs that control and regulate how they function.

PART 1: LIGHT AND YOUR CIRCADIAN RHYTHM

Both circadian light and UV light can be very helpful for sleep, healing, and longevity.

You have heard us preach over and over about how important it is to get good sleep. Getting at least eight hours of restful sleep can be a key to weight loss, mental clarity, and so much more. One of the best ways to ensure a good night of sleep is to get your circadian clock in rhythm and get your body to naturally produce melatonin at the right times.

Our eyes have a receptor that responds to the presence of light—specifically blue light—and signals the SCN (suprachiasmatic nucleus) in the brain. The activation of the SCN (due to the presence of blue light in the eye) prevents the pineal gland from producing melatonin, the hormone that signals drowsiness and sleep. A lack of blue light in the eye signals the pineal gland to produce melatonin, inducing drowsiness and natural sleep cycles.

It is critical to support this process to enable good sleep cycles. There are two ways to do so:

- **Get twenty minutes of sunlight within two hours of waking.** Go outside and face the sun. (If you wear glasses or contacts, take them off.) Don't look directly at the sun, but let the blue light hit your eyes and start your circadian clock. Get twenty minutes of light exposure to stimulate your SCN and energize you for the day ahead. If you can, also remove some clothing so that your skin absorbs some UV light to energize your body, stimulate the manufacture of vitamin D, and generate cholesterol sulfates, which improve moods and boost the health of your cells.

- **Limit exposure to blue light at bedtime.** Exposure to blue light contributes to poor sleep cycles. Interior lighting, smartphones, computers, and TVs all emit blue light that inhibits the pineal gland from producing melatonin in a natural cycle. If you plan to continue to use these kinds of devices or watch TV in the evening, invest in a pair of blue-blocking glasses. They block all the blue light so you can watch TV, use your devices, and so on while allowing your brain and pineal gland to naturally produce melatonin at the right time to promote sleep. Your bedtime will dictate when you should start wearing the glasses; we recommend putting them on three to four hours before bed.

These two things—getting direct sunlight in the morning and blocking blue light in the evening—are the most important things you can do to improve your sleep and overall health.

The UV light and infrared light that you're exposed to also assist with many processes in your body. We know how important vitamin D is for moods, strong bones, cholesterol, and many health processes (see Chapter 2). You might be getting 5,000 IU of vitamin D3 from a supplement, but you can make 1,000 IU per minute of being in a bright, sunny location with your skin exposed. So in just thirty minutes, you can get 30,000 IU! As is so often the case, the traditional thinking about the harmfulness of commonsense UV light exposure is wrong. Yes, third-degree sunburns are harmful. However, UV light in moderate doses is not harmful; in fact, it can be very beneficial.

PART 2: WATER

We often discuss the importance of drinking enough water. When we say to drink half your body weight in ounces each day, we really mean it. As far as cellular health is concerned, spring water is your best choice; it doesn't contain all the chlorine and fluoride found in

ADJUST YOUR DEVICE SETTINGS

This technique of blocking blue light is becoming more mainstream. Even iOS devices (such as the iPhone and iPad) now have a setting to limit blue light in the morning and evening. Just go to Settings, choose Display & Brightness, and enable Night Shift. Set it to the warmest setting, which limits the blue light coming from the device. We have ours set to turn on at 6 to 7 p.m., depending on the time of year.

city and municipal water supplies. When choosing a spring water source, there are online tools to help you find local sources, such as findaspring.com.

PART 3: GROUNDING

The earth has a negative charge. We have long known that having a slightly alkaline body is associated with many health benefits, including lower rates of cancer, better sleep, and reduced inflammation. When you connect to the earth through an electrical ground, you negatively charge your body; in other words, you make it more alkaline. Today, most of us are isolated from the earth by our homes and cars—and thus we don't enjoy these benefits.

The best way to ground yourself is to wear rubber grounding shoes. A section of the shoe conducts electricity, grounding you to the earth as you walk. There are many versions out there, depending on your style preferences—or you can just go barefoot!

Another option is to use a grounding mat, which plugs into a standard electrical outlet; modern outlets have an earth ground (the round hole at the bottom). You can use a grounding mat at your computer, in bed, or anywhere you spend a lot of time.

CHECKLIST FOR ACCELERATING HEALING AND WEIGHT LOSS

Everyone is different when it comes to weight loss. No two bodies are the same. We have covered a lot of information in this book, so we've made a checklist to help you be as successful as possible in your keto lifestyle.

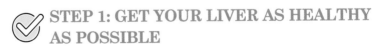 ## STEP 1: GET YOUR LIVER AS HEALTHY AS POSSIBLE

The liver performs more than 400 different jobs and is the body's most important metabolism-enhancing organ; it acts as a filter to clear the body of toxins, metabolize protein, control hormone balance, and enhance your immune system. Your liver might be to blame if you are on edge, easily stressed, have elevated cholesterol, skin irritations, depression, sleep difficulties, indigestion, kidney damage, brain fog, hypothyroidism, chronic fatigue, weight gain, poor memory, PMS, blood sugar imbalances, or allergies. The liver also plays a role in migraines; if this vital organ is overloaded with toxic substances, it can cause inflammation that triggers migraine pain. If you have tried many ways to improve your health and energy level and nothing has helped, your tired liver might be triggering your difficulties. Restoring your liver function is one of the most essential actions you can take for your health. When the liver gets congested, it will remain that way and get worse until it is cleaned and revitalized.

Your liver is a worker bee that can even regenerate its own damaged cells! However, it is not invincible. When your liver is abused, lacks essential nutrients, or is overwhelmed by toxins, it no longer performs as it should. Fat can build up in the liver and just under the skin, hormone imbalances can develop, and toxin levels can increase and get into the bloodstream. The liver metabolizes fats, proteins, and carbohydrates for fuel. It breaks down amino acids from proteins into various pieces to help build muscle, which directly affects your calorie burn.

The liver delivers amino acids to the bloodstream for hormone balance, a critical task that helps your body avoid water retention, bloating, cravings, and other undesirable weight-related issues. Amino acids also help move waste, such as damaged cholesterol, used estrogen, and insulin to the liver for detoxification and elimination through the kidneys. The liver's most important function—and the one that puts it at the greatest risk for damage—is to detoxify the numerous toxins that attack our bodies every day.

A healthy liver works with the lungs, kidneys, skin, and intestines, detoxifying many damaging substances and eliminating them without polluting the bloodstream. Cleaning your liver and eating the right foods improves liver metabolism, and you start burning fat instead of glucose. As your liver function improves, so does your energy level.

With more energy, fitness improves because you can exercise more and improve your muscle tone. The liver will naturally cleanse itself if you stop putting chemicals in your mouth and on your skin. You can speed up liver cleansing with milk thistle and

Healing Your Liver

- Stop using topical chemicals.
- Eliminate sources of obesogens, such as dryer sheets and scented candles.
- Eliminate fructose from your diet.
- Stop drinking alcohol.
- Eat foods that contain cholesterol.

Get Your Liver
Enzymes Checked

Elevated liver enzymes can make it difficult for you to lose weight and/or can cause poor moods. Elevated liver enzymes can also create problems with your liver function and can result in high cholesterol numbers.

sweating. Sit in a sauna or practice hot yoga (yoga done in a hot room to induce sweating). Just make sure to hydrate and refuel your electrolytes afterward!

The liver affects our bodies in many ways:

- The liver is where T4 is converted to T3 (the activated thyroid hormone).
- Excess estrogen blocks production of T3. T4 needs to be converted to activated T3, a process that happens in the liver. T3 is what makes us feel good. EstroFactors helps detox this bad estrogen from the liver, which in turn heals the liver and increases T3 production.
- If it is not tired and toxic, the liver breaks down fat.
- This important organ not only helps you lose weight, but also controls your moods.
- If you do not consume enough cholesterol, your liver will make the rest, which keeps the liver in overdrive.

STEP 2: CUT OUT ALL DAIRY (EVEN LOW-CARB, HIGH-FAT DAIRY)

We are typical natives of Wisconsin. We love our cheese, and we even wear cheeseheads when we watch the Green Bay Packers play football. No lie, we own four cheeseheads. However, we also know that consuming dairy prevents many of our clients from reaching their goals. We've found that cutting out all dairy helps many clients get to their goal weight. So, while writing this book, our family cut out dairy for a while. We skipped the butter, cream, cheese, yogurt, and whey.

When you have a damaged and inflamed gut, a phenomenon called "atrophy of the villi" occurs. Your body digests dairy at the ends of the villi. If cutting out dairy seems too daunting to do forever, eliminate dairy for 30 days; once you heal your intestinal wall with an anti-inflammatory ketogenic diet, you can try to incorporate dairy foods again (in smaller doses at first). At the end of the 30 days, weigh yourself, eat some lactose-free dairy such as ghee, and then weigh yourself at the same time the following day. If you are heavier, don't panic; it's not actual fat gain. Instead, you are retaining water. If you do retain water, we suggest skipping all dairy for two months and then testing again. If you don't retain water, then you can reincorporate dairy into your diet. If weight loss stalls at any point, try removing dairy again.

 ## STEP 3: LIMIT VARIETY ON YOUR PLATE

Studies show when you eat the same food, the reward signaling in the brain decreases with each bite, which means you are less likely to overeat.[1] However, a lot of variety allows you to change up flavors, which increases the likelihood that you will overeat. This is one reason why a buffet is a recipe for disaster. You can take a couple of bites of many different flavors, which means you keep moving on to the next flavor and overeat. Smell and taste combine to make overeating easy when we are eating at a potluck or buffet because there are so many choices to keep stimulating the senses. However, if you have one food on your plate, your brain gets bored and sends a signal to stop eating.

 ## STEP 4: CUT OUT ALCOHOL

Eliminating alcohol is very important for sleep, moods, and metabolism. Alcohol does not help you get into ketosis; if anything, alcohol is holding you back from being your best self—not just physically but also mentally.

 ## STEP 5: ELIMINATE ALL VEGETABLE AND SEED OILS

Look at packaged foods, including marinara sauces—most use canola, cottonseed, soybean, or corn oil. Even "healthy" mayonnaise, salad dressings, and roasted nuts are most likely made with vegetable oils. Omega-6 vegetable and seed oils are very inflammatory.

 ## STEP 6: DETOX BAD ESTROGEN

Do not microwave in plastic or drink from plastic water bottles. Eliminate non-organic foods laced with synthetic estrogen. Eliminate obesogens (chemicals that disrupt normal development) in things such as dryer sheets and synthetic fragrances because they increase estrogen in both women and men.

WHEY-FREE PROTEIN POWDER

Cutting out dairy means no whey protein, either. Jay Robb, our favorite brand of protein powders, makes a tasty egg white protein and a quality beef protein powder.

STEP 7: AVOID PLASTICS

Plastics are estrogenic; that is, they produce compounds that stimulate bad estrogens. Avoid heating food on plastic plates in the microwave, putting hot food on plastic plates, or putting hot drinks in plastic cups. Avoid bottled water, too, because the heat from the semi-trailers in which the water is shipped causes estrogen to leach into the water.

 STEP 8: GO NUMBER TWO EVERY DAY

If you don't poop, estrogens get reabsorbed and locked into your fat cells.

 STEP 9: BENEFIT FROM THE AFTERBURN EFFECT

Wait a little while after a hard workout to eat. When you work out, you increase the human growth hormone, which stimulates the production of ketones. The afterburn effect can stimulate up to 400 more calories if you wait to eat. Being keto-adapted allows you to keep burning fat for fuel rather than cannibalizing muscle like a sugar burner would. Once you eat, your fast is broken.

 STEP 10: NO SNACKING

If you are constantly fueling your body and increasing insulin, you cannot get into the fat-burning mode. Do not eat every two hours.

 STEP 11: GET ENOUGH SLEEP

Get at least eight hours of quality sleep every night!

 STEP 12: EAT SLOWLY

Eating slowly lowers the insulin response and helps register the hormone leptin, which gives your body the signal that you are full. One way to ensure that you eat slowly is to chew thirty-two times before swallowing. Food should be liquid before you swallow it.

STEP 13: WATCH WHAT AND WHEN YOU DRINK

First, don't drink your calories. Drinking your calories doesn't register leptin (the I'm full signal) as well as chewing whole foods. As a result you consume a lot more calories a lot quicker than you would if chewing. Just eat real, whole foods.

Also, don't drink while you're eating. Liquids dilute your digestive enzymes. Stop drinking about thirty to sixty minutes before meals, and wait for about thirty to sixty minutes after eating before drinking any liquids. If you're taking pre-meal supplements, take them with only as much water as you need to get them down.

STEP 14: STAY HYDRATED

Drinking half your body weight in ounces helps both the kidneys and the liver. When your kidneys are dehydrated, the liver stops its main jobs and helps out the kidneys. When you are well hydrated, the liver can focus on burning fat. Be nice to your liver, people! Your mitochondria are primarily made up of water and rely on a sufficient supply of water to ensure proper function.

STEP 15: DECREASE STRESS

If you hate your job, it's time to find a new one that helps you embrace this new lifestyle. We realize this is easier said than done, but you spend most of your time at your job; make it something you look forward to doing every day. We had one client quit his job to become a fitness instructor. Man, he looks like a new person!

Exercise is a stressor, too. Don't plan on running a marathon in the middle of a divorce or after a death in the family. During a stressful time in your life, yoga is a better fit.

Evaluate relationships that are causing too much stress. Are some people in your life toxic and trying to demolish your health goals? It might be time to find more supportive people to associate with.

STEP 16: DECREASE STRESSFUL EATING SITUATIONS

Do you often have lunch meetings at the office? Do you notice that you get indigestion or diarrhea after a stressful eating situation such as this? When you are under stress, your heart rate goes up, your blood pressure rises, and blood is forced away from your digestive system and moved to your legs, arms, and head for quick thinking. During stressful times, there can be as much as four times less blood flowing to your digestive system, which causes your metabolism to be sluggish and your body not to burn those calories as effectively. In that state, proper digestion entirely shuts down.

Keep the meetings at work and enjoy a little peaceful break for lunch. Also, try not to eat while stressed after an argument; instead, try yoga for exercise; the blood flow is going to your extremities anyway!

 ## STEP 17: ADD HERBS AND SPICES TO YOUR MEALS

We love to hide herbs and spices in meatloaf, meatballs, chili, and spaghetti sauce. To make life even easier, try our Maria's Keto Kitchen spice mixes, available at keto-adapted.com/keto-spices/!

 ## STEP 18: CHANGE YOUR SKINCARE AND TOPICAL PRODUCTS

Your liver can become congested not only from the foods you eat but also from the soaps, makeup, and other products you use on your skin. We had one client whose liver enzymes returned to normal after she ditched all the lotions and makeup she was using!

 ## STEP 19: STEER CLEAR OF FLUORIDE

Get rid of all the fluoride and chlorine in your body. Many fruits, veggies, and other crops grown in the United States are sprayed with cryolite, a pesticide that contains a high amount of energy-zapping fluoride. Today, Americans consume four times the amount of fluoride than they did in 1940, the year it began to be added to drinking water to prevent cavities. It is found in many commercial products, including soup, soda, and black tea. Even the U.S. Centers for Disease Control (CDC) has expressed concern that more than 200 million Americans are exposed to extreme levels of fluoride.[2] In addition, too much fluoride wreaks havoc on our thyroids.

 ## STEP 20: LIMIT EATING OUT

When did it become so common to eat out? We remember when eating out was a rare Friday-night treat. Now, if you walk into a restaurant during the lunch hour, it is packed! Too often we hear complaints about the cost of eating healthy when in reality eating out is way more expensive. We went to brunch the other day with our boys, and we all ordered eggs and salmon with extra hollandaise, a side of chorizo, and a side of bacon. Craig got an organic coffee, Maria and the boys drank water. The bill was $63! For eggs! Furthermore, you can never be sure which cooking oils restaurants are using. Most likely they are using inflammatory vegetable oils. Gluten and dairy also sneak in and can cause inflammation; even meats are often marinated in soy sauce, which contains gluten.

 ## STEP 21: STOP THE NEGATIVE SELF-TALK

Tell yourself that you can do it. Think positively and surround yourself with positive people who will support you on your journey. Even an online support group can help you stay on course with the keto diet.

WHY WEIGHT LOSS GETS HARDER

It probably won't come as a surprise to hear that losing weight gets harder each time you attempt a diet. The liver is the main organ that governs fat loss. It processes hormones, cleanses the cells of toxins, makes cholesterol, breaks down fats, and metabolizes carbohydrates and proteins, along with handling many other bodily functions. When your liver is constantly stressed by dieting, it gets tired and toxic, which makes it unable to assist you in losing weight. In traditional Chinese medicine, liver function is believed to govern our emotions. When your liver is stressed by poor food, alcohol, fructose, sugar, lack of sleep, or pollution, you are most likely to be depressed, anxious, or angry. Low liver function causes food cravings, binge eating, and excretion of too much cortisol, which causes more liver stress. It's a vicious cycle! Also, if you go on antidepressants because your liver is causing low moods, the antidepressant causes more toxicity to your liver, which causes more depression and inability to lose weight.

The term "leaky gut" refers to when waste and partially digested foods are allowed into the bloodstream because of perforations in the intestinal wall. People who are very sensitive to food poisoning have weak intestinal walls that allow bacteria to enter the blood easily. Antacids allow food particles to sit in your digestive system too long, causing stress on the intestinal wall and leaving you subject to leaky gut, water retention, and stress on the liver. Leaky gut can cause some people to gain 10 to 15 pounds of extra fluids. A healthy body is about two-thirds water (hydrated cells are happy cells!), but when you have a leaky gut, water gets trapped and is unable to filter out toxins and waste, which also inhibits cell functions. Your lymphatic system gets overwhelmed, which causes undesired cellulite to form.

Also, your body and fat cells want to stay at homeostasis (maintain their current state). When you lose weight, your fat cells shrink. When this happens, one of the twenty-five messengers (hormones) in the fat cells sends powerful messages to the brain to eat, often sending you into an overfeeding binge, making the fat cells even larger, which makes your weight set point even higher. Yo-yo dieting is very detrimental to fat cell growth.

The liver ensures proper hormone balance. We often see estrogen dominance in many of our clients. Estrogen dominance happens because we are exposed to unhealthy external estrogen, such as non-organic meat and milk, alcohol, fructose, microwaving in plastics, drinking from plastic water bottles, and eating flax or soy. Even soap leaches estrogens into the blood. However, estrogens are detoxed by a healthy liver. Disruptions in detoxification contribute to estrogen dominance, which causes difficulty in losing belly fat. Hormone balance is important for helping enable weight loss. Insulin, estrogen, testosterone, leptin, ghrelin, glucagon, thyroid, progesterone, cortisol, human growth hormone, as well as other hormones determine our rate of fat metabolism, cravings, energy, and sleep.

The liver is also responsible for more than half of your body's cholesterol production. Most of this cholesterol is used to produce bile, which breaks down fat. Bile gets stored in the gallbladder and is used to digest food; bile salts stimulate the secretion of water into the large intestine, which helps us with proper bowel movements. One sign of a tired liver is that you don't have a daily bowel movement. Other signs are excess belly fat, fatty cysts, and age spots.

Following are some signs of liver stress:

- Low T3 production (T4 is converted to activated T3 in the liver, not the thyroid)
- Chronic indigestion
- Constipation
- Cellulite
- PMS or menopausal symptoms
- Low moods—depression, anxiety, and irritability
- Muscle or joint pain
- Headaches or migraines
- Exhaustion

The good news is that the liver can heal rapidly when provided the right nutrients. A well-formulated ketogenic diet that omits processed foods makes this possible.

WHAT TO DO AFTER A CHEAT

Almost every day, a client asks us, "I cheated. Now what?" Maria especially has a heavy heart when she hears this because at one point in her life, Fridays meant cheat time.

You are not defined by what the scale says or the size of your jeans! You are defined by your individuality. The choices you make today create habits that have consequences—consequences that you have to face up to and live with every day. You can make good choices that make you stronger, or you can make bad choices that fulfill you for only a moment and then leave you feeling ill and unhappy for days—or maybe even years—afterward.

I lived in denial for too long. All of my friends ate ice cream and chips and didn't have weight problems. I wanted to live like that, too. However, it wasn't just my outward appearance that depressed me. I didn't feel strong and energized while eating those foods. I always despised how awful I felt after I cheated. Journaling about it helped me remember that feeling and put a stop to my bad eating habits.

It is easy to fall prey to peer pressure about the "normal" way to eat. We struggled with it, too, but over time, we overcame that pressure. We can't eat "normal" anymore, and we don't want to be "normal" anyway. We want to be Maria and Craig.

Here are some tips to help you avoid cheat days:

- **Accept and forgive yourself.** Be aware of what happened; do not live in denial. Accept the choice that you made and forgive yourself for it.
- **Keep a journal.** Remember how awesome you feel when you are sticking to the keto lifestyle and journal how you feel after a cheat.
- **Remember that change will come.** When you change the bad habit, the outcome also will change, even if it takes time.
- **Remember that keto is a lifestyle.** Eating keto isn't a diet for us; it's a lifestyle. We love food, and we will always love food, but more importantly, we love the way we feel when we eat like this! (And yes, we enjoy a keto dessert every day!) That's why Maria loves creating delicious recipes that make people love to eat keto. We want you to be able to do this with ease!

IN CLOSING

With all this information in hand, we wish you luck in your journey to a healthy weight. We know all this might seem overwhelming and foreign, but try one new thing each week, and eventually you'll reach your goal. This week, maybe change your breakfast from cereal to eggs. Next week, maybe start walking after dinner. Baby steps are what worked for us. Instead of feeling overwhelmed, feel empowered by having the tools you need to succeed. No more deprivation diets consisting of fat-free, man-made foods. Eat real food, get real satisfaction, and achieve a healthy metabolism.

If you are like us and you are more of a visual learner, or you want more information about what we do, we offer many Skype and online video classes at http://mariamindbodyhealth.com/video-classes/. We also offer lots of support options on our subscription site, keto-adapted.com.

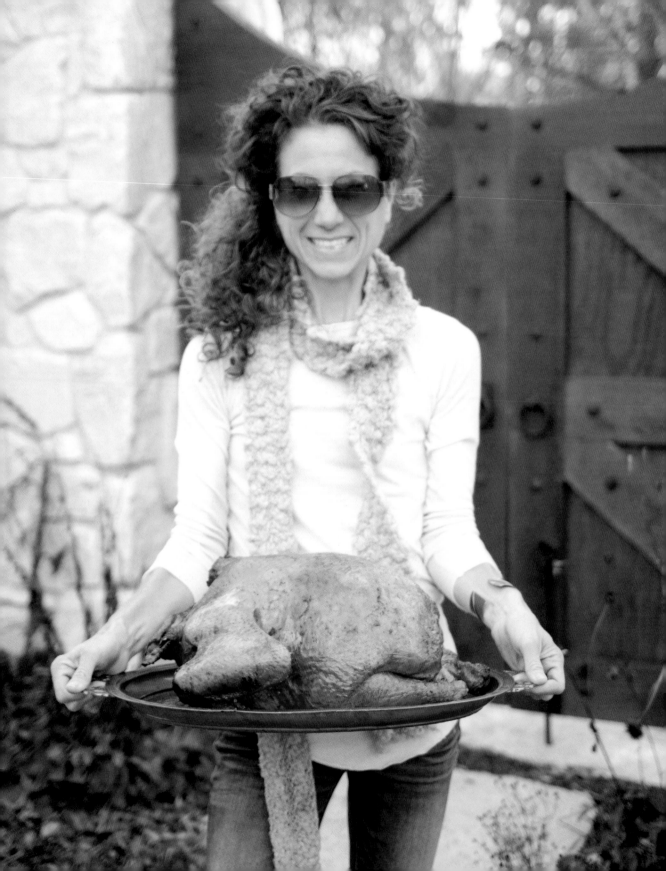

END NOTES

CHAPTER 1

1. U.S. Food and Drug Administration (FDA) data.

2. Lou, You-Rong, Qing-Yun Peng, Tao Li, Christopher Medvecky, Yong Lin, Weichung Joe Shih, Allan Conney, et al. "Effects of High-Fat Diets Rich in Either Omega-3 or Omega-6 Fatty Acids on UVB-Induced Skin Carcinogenesis in SKH-1 Mice." *Carcinogenesis* 32, no. 7 (2011): 1078–1084, www.ncbi.nlm.nih.gov/pmc/articles/PMC3128560/.

3. "Cellular sweet spot found in skin-cancer battle." *ScienceDaily* website, June 12, 2017, www.sciencedaily.com/releases/2017/06/170612124420.htm.

4. Taubes, Gary. *The Case Against Sugar.* New York: Alfred A. Knopf, 2016.

5. Taubes, Gary. *Why We Get Fat and What to Do About It.* New York, Alfred A. Knopf, 2011.

6. Crowe, Kelly. "Sugar Industry's Secret Documents Echo Tobacco Tactics." CBC News, March 8, 2013, www.cbc.ca/news/health/sugar-industry-s-secret-documents-echo-tobacco-tactics-1.1369231.

7. Domonoske, Camila. "50 Years Ago, Sugar Industry Quietly Paid Scientists to Point Blame at Fat." NPR website, September 13, 2016. www.npr.org/sections/thetwo-way/2016/09/13/493739074/50-years-ago-sugar-industry-quietly-paid-scientists-to-point-blame-at-fat.

8. Kearns, Cristin E., Laura A. Schmidt, and Stanton A. Glantz. "Sugar Industry and Coronary Heart Disease Research: A Historical Analysis of Internal Industry Documents." *JAMA Internal Medicine* 176, no. 11 (2016): 1680–1685, http://jamanetwork.com/journals/jamainternalmedicine/article-abstract/2548255.

9. O'Connor, Anahad. "How the Sugar Industry Shifted Blame to Fat." *The New York Times*, September 12, 2016, https://mobile.nytimes.com/2016/09/13/well/eat/how-the-sugar-industry-shifted-blame-to-fat.html.

10. Cohen, Rich. "Sugar Love (A Not So Sweet Story)." *National Geographic*, August 2013, http://ngm.nationalgeographic.com/2013/08/sugar/cohen-text?rptregcta=join_free_np&rptregcampaign=20130722_lightbox_membership_nonhp_all_1#close-modal.

11. Bridger, Tracey. "Childhood obesity and cardiovascular disease." *Paediatrics & Child Health* 14, no.3 (2009), www.ncbi.nlm.nih.gov/pmc/articles/PMC2690549/.

12. Arcidiacono, Biagio, Stefania Iiritano, Aurora Nocera, Katiuscia Possidente, Maria Nevolo, Valeria Ventura, Daniela Foti, et al. "Insulin Resistance and Cancer Risk: An Overview of the Pathogenetic Mechanisms." *Experimental Diabetes Research*, 2012, www.hindawi.com/journals/jdr/2012/789174/.

13. Zhou, Weihua, Purna Mukherjee, Michael A. Kiebish, William T. Markis, John G. Mantis, and Thomas N. Seyfried. "The Calorically Restricted Ketogenic Diet, an Effective Alternative Therapy for Malignant Brain Cancer." *Nutrition & Metabolism*, February 2007, https://nutritionandmetabolism.biomedcentral.com/articles/10.1186/1743-7075-4-5.

14. Poff, Angela M., Csilla Ari, Thomas N. Seyfried, and Dominic P. D'Agostino. "The Ketogenic Diet and Hyperbaric Oxygen Therapy Prolong Survival in Mice with Systemic Metastatic Cancer." *PLOS One*, June 2013, http://journals.plos.org/plosone/article/file?id=10.1371/journal.pone.0065522&type=printable.

CHAPTER 2

1. Knutson, Kristin L., Karine Spiegel, Plamen Panev, and Eve Van Cauter. "The Metabolic Consequences of Sleep Deprivation." *Sleep Medicine Reviews* 11, no. 3 (2007): 163–178, www.ncbi.nlm.nih.gov/pmc/articles/PMC1991337/.

2. Kim, Jong In, Jin Young Huh, Jee Hyran Sohn, Sung Sik Choe, Yun Sok Lee, Chun Yan Lim, Ala Jo, et al. "Lipid-Overloaded Enlarged Adipocytes Provoke Insulin Resistance Independent of Inflammation." *Molecular and Cellular Biology* 35, no. 10 (2015.): 1686–1699, http://mcb.asm.org/content/35/10/1686.full.

3. Dave Feldman. *Cholesterol Code: Reverse Engineering the Mystery* website, accessed November 10, 2017, http://cholesterolcode.com/.

4. Jacobs, Peter C., Martijn J. A. Gondrie, Yolanda van der Graaf, Harry J. de Koning, Ivana Isgum, Bram van Ginnekin, and Willem P. T. M. Mali. "Coronary Artery Calcium Can Predict All-Cause Mortality and Cardiovascular Events on Low-Dose CT Screening for Lung Cancer." *American Journal of Roentgenology*, 198 (2011): 505–511, www.ajronline.org/doi/pdf/10.2214/AJR.10.5577.

5. Cummins, Ivor. "Dr. Joseph R. Kraft—Stories from the World War II Era—Part I." Video. August 20, 2016, www.thefatemperor.com/blog/2016/8/20/dr-joseph-r-kraft-stories-from-the-world-war-ii-era-part-1?rq=kraft.

6. Enzinger, C., F. Fazekas, P. M. Matthews, S. Ropele, H. Schmidt, S. Smith, and R. Schmidt. "Risk Factors for Progression of Brain Atrophy in Aging." *Neurology* 65, no. 10 (2005: 1704-1711, www.ncbi.nlm.nih.gov/pubmed/15911795.

7. Shishehbor, Mehdi H., Byron J. Hoogwerf, and Michael S. Lauer. "Association of Triglyceride-to-HDL Cholesterol Ratio with Heart Rate Recovery." *Diabetes Care* 27, no. 4 (2004): 936–941, http://care.diabetesjournals.org/content/27/4/936.

8. He, Congcong, Rhea Sumpter, Jr., and Beth Levine. "Exercise Induces Autophagy in Peripheral Tissues and in the Brain." *Autophagy* 8, no. 10 (2012): 1548–1551. www.ncbi.nlm.nih.gov/pmc/articles/PMC3463459/.

9. Lindqvist, P. G., E. Epstein, M. Landin-Olsson, C. Ingvar, M. Stenbeck, and H. Olsson. "Avoidance of Sun Exposure Is a Risk Factor for All-Cause Mortality: Results from the Melanoma in Southern Sweden Cohort." *Journal of Internal Medicine*, 276, no. 1 (2014): 77–86, www.ncbi.nlm.nih.gov/pubmed/24697969.

10. Thompson, Dennis. "Skin Cancer Could Be Hiding Where You'd Never Expect: The Sole of Your Foot." CBS News website, HealthDay, June 16, 2016, www.cbsnews.com/news/skin-cancer-melanoma-body-parts-sole-of-foot/.

11. Westerdahl, Johan, Christian Ingvar, Anna Måsbäck, and Håkan Olsson. "Sunscreen Use and Malignant Melanoma." *International Journal of Cancer* 87, no. 1 (2000): 145–150, http://onlinelibrary.wiley.com/doi/10.1002/1097-0215(20000701)87:1%3C145::AID-IJC22%3E3.0.CO;2-3/full.

CHAPTER 3

1. Pinckaers, Philippe J. M., Tyler A. Churchward-Venne, David Bailey, and Luc J. C. van Loon. "Ketone Bodies and Exercise Performance: The Next Magic Bullet or Merely Hype?" *Sports Medicine*, 47, no. 3 (2016): 383–391, www.ncbi.nlm.nih.gov/pmc/articles/PMC5309297/.

2. CDC Report, *Health, United States,* 2015, www.cdc.gov/nchs/data/hus/hus15.pdf#056.

3. Dietary Guidelines for Americans, 2010, www.health.gov/dietaryguidelines/dga2010/dietaryguidelines2010.pdf.

4. Cronise, Raymond J., David A. Sinclair, and Andrew A. Bremer. "Oxidative Priority, Meal Frequency, and the Energy Economy of Food and Activity: Implications for Longevity, Obesity and Cardiometabolic Disease." *Metabolic Syndrome Related Disorders* 15, no. 1 (2017): 6–17, www.ncbi.nlm.nih.gov/pmc/articles/PMC5326984/.

5. Ibid.

6. Heinbecker, Peter. "Studies on the Metabolism of Eskimos." *Journal of Biological Chemistry* 80 (1928): 461–475, www.jbc.org./content/80/2/461.short.

7. Foster-Schubert, K. E., J. Overduin, C. E. Prudom, J. Liu, H. S. Callahan, B. D. Gaylinn, M. O. Thorner, et al. "Acyl and Total Ghrelin Are Suppressed Strongly by Ingested Proteins, Weakly by Lipids,

and Biphasically by Carbohydrates." *Journal of Clinical Endocrinology & Metabolism* 93, no. 5 (2008): 1971–1979, https://academic.oup.com/jcem/article/93/5/1971/2599032/Acyl-and-Total-Ghrelin-Are-Suppressed-Strongly-by.

8. Hellerstein, M. K., R. A. Neese, and J. M. Schwarz. "Model for Measuring Absolute Rates of Hepatic De Novo Lipogenesis and Reesterification of Free Fatty Acids." *American Journal of Physiology–Endocrinology and Metabolism* 265, no. 5 (1993): E814–E820. http://ajpendo.physiology.org/content/265/5/E814

9. Reshef, Lea, Yael Olswang, Hanoch Cassuto, Barak Blum, Colleen M. Croniger, Satish C. Kalhan, Shirley M. Tilghman, et al. "Glyceroneogenesis and the Triglyceride/Fatty Acid Cycle," *Journal of Biological Chemistry* 278 (2003): 30413–30416, http://www.jbc.org/content/278/33/30413.full.

10. Frayn, Keith N., Peter Arner, and Hannele Yki-Järvinen. "Fatty Acid Metabolism in Adipose Tissue, Muscle and Liver in Health and Disease," *Essays in Biochemistry* 42 (2006): 89–103, http://essays.biochemistry.org/content/42/89.

CHAPTER 4

1. Ahola-Erkkilä, S., C. J. Carroll, K. Peltola-Mjösund, V. Tulkki, I. Mattila, T. Seppänen-Laakso, M. Oresic, et al. "Ketogenic Diet Slows Down Mitochondrial Myopathy Progression in Mice," *Human Molecular Genetics* 19, no. 10 (2010): 1974–1984, www.ncbi.nlm.nih.gov/pubmed/20167576.

2. Phinney, S. D., E. S. Horton, E. A. Sims, J. S. Hanson, E. Danforth Jr., and B. M. LaGrange. "Capacity for Moderate Exercise in Obese Subjects After Adaptation to a Hypocaloric, Ketogenic Diet," *Journal of Clinical Investigation* 66, no. 5 (1980): 1152–1161, www.ncbi.nlm.nih.gov/pubmed/7000826.

3. Bikman, Benjamin. "Insulin vs. Ketones—The Battle for Brown Fat." Insulin IQ video lecture, 34:33. March 18, 2017. www.insuliniq.com/dr-bikman-addresses-worlds-foremost-lchf-authorities-at-breckenridge-2017-conference/.

4. Cahill, George F., Jr. "Fuel Metabolism in Starvation." *Annual Review of Nutrition* 26 (2006): 1–22, http://ltc-ead.nutes.ufrj.br/constructore/objetos/Art%206-M%F3dulo%201.pdf.

5. O'Donnell, Martin, Salim Yusuf, Andrew Mente, Peggy Gao, Johannes F. Mann, Koon Teo, Matthew McQueen, et al. "Urinary Sodium and Potassium Excretion and Risk of Cardiovascular Events." *Journal of American Medical Association* 306, no. 20 (2011): 2229–2238, jama.jamanetwork.com/article.aspx?articleid=1105553.

CHAPTER 5

1. "Mechanism of Action and Physiologic Effects of Thyroid Hormones," *Thyroid and Parathyroid Glands* website, accessed November 6, 2017, www.vivo.colostate.edu/hbooks/pathphys/endocrine/thyroid/physio.html.

2. Godfrey, R. J., Z. Madgwick, and G. P. Whyte. "The Exercise-Induced Growth Hormone Response in Athletes." *Sports Medicine* 33, no. 8 (2003): 599–613, www.ncbi.nlm.nih.gov/pubmed/12797841.

3. "Why Lost Weight Can Creep Back On," *BBC News Health* website, December 2, 2005, http://news.bbc.co.uk/2/hi/health/4487690.stm.

4. Rosenbaum, M., E. M. Murphy, S. B. Heymsfield, D. E. Matthews, and R. L. Liebl. "Low Dose Leptin Administration Reverses Effects of Sustained Weight-Reduction on Energy Expenditure and Circulating Concentrations of Thyroid Hormones." *Journal of Clinical Endocrinology & Metabolism* 87, no. 5 (2002): 2391–2394, www.ncbi.nlm.nih.gov/pubmed/11994393.

5. Rosenbaum, M., R. Goldsmith, D. Bloomfield, A. Magnano, L. Weimer, S. Heymsfield, D. Gallagher, et al. "Low-Dose Leptin Reverses Skeletal Muscle, Autonomic, and Neuroendocrine Adaptations to Maintenance of Reduced Weight." *Journal of Clinical Investigation* 115, no. 12 (2005): 3579–3586, www.ncbi.nlm.nih.gov/pmc/articles/PMC1297250/.

6. Batterham, R. L., M. A. Cohen, S. M. Ellis, C. W. LeRoux, D. J. Withers, G. S. Frost, M. A. Ghatei, et

al. "Inhibition of Food Intake in Obese Subjects by Peptide YY3–36." *New England Journal of Medicine* 349, no. 10 (2003): 941–948, www.nejm.org/doi/full/10.1056/NEJMoa030204#t=article

7. Colburn, Theo, Dianne Dumanoski, and John Peterson Meyers. *Our Stolen Future: Are We Threatening Our Fertility, Intelligence, and Survival? A Scientific Detective Story.* New York: Plume, 1997.

8. Mulligan, T., M. F. Frick, Q. C. Zuraw, A. Stemhagen, and C. McWhirter. "Prevalence of Hypogonadism in Males Aged at Least 45 Years: The HIM Study." *International Journal of Clinical Practice* 60, no. 7 (2006): 762–769, www.ncbi.nlm.nih.gov/pubmed/16846397?dopt=AbstractPlus.

9. Maggio, M., F. Lauretani, F. DeVita, S. Basaria, G. Lippi, V. Buttò, M. Luci, et al. "Multiple Hormonal Dysregulation as Determinant of Low Physical Performance and Mobility in Older Persons." *Current Pharmaceutical Design* 20, no. 19 (2014): 3119–3148, www.ncbi.nlm.nih.gov/pmc/articles/PMC5155505/.

CHAPTER 6

1. Tjonneland, A., K. Overvad, M. M. Bergmann, G. Nagel, J. Linseisen, G. Hallmans, R. Palmqvist, et al. "Linoleic Acid, a Dietary N-6 Polyunsaturated Fatty Acid, and the Aetiology of ulcerative Colitis: A Nested Case-Control Study within a European Prospective Cohort Study." *Gut* 58, no. 12 (2009): 1606–1611, www.ncbi.nlm.nih.gov/pubmed/19628674.

2. Perheentupa, J. and K. Raivio. "Fructose-Induced Hyperuricaemia." *The Lancet* 2, no. 7515 (1967): 528-531, www.ncbi.nlm.nih.gov/pubmed/4166890.

3. Tolmunen, T., J. Hintikka, A. Ruusunen, S. Voutilainen, A. Tanskanen, V. P. Valkonen, H. Viinamäki, et al. "Dietary Folate and the Risk of Depression in Finnish Middle-Aged Men: A Prospective Follow-Up Study." *Psychotherapy and Pschosomatics* 73, no. 6 (2004): 334–339, www.ncbi.nlm.nih.gov/pubmed/15479987.

4. Harley, Kim and Kimberly Parra. HERMOSA Study, 2016. https://cerch.berkeley.edu/research-programs/hermosa-study.

5. Yang, Yu-Xiao, James Lewis, Solomon Epstein, and David Metz. "Long-Term Proton Pump Inhibitor Therapy and Risk of Hip Fracture." *Journal of the American Medical Association* 296, no. 24 (2006): 2947–2953, https://jamanetwork.com/journals/jama/fullarticle/204783.

6. Feilden, Tom. "Osteoporosis Drugs May Make Bones Weaker." BBC News Health, March 1, 2017, www.bbc.com/news/health-39122541.

7. Kumar, Vijay, Manoj Rajadhyaksha, and Jacobo Wortsman. "Celiac Disease–Associated Autoimmune Endocrinopathies." *Clinical and Vaccine Immunology* 8, no. 4 (2001): 678–685, http://cvi.asm.org/content/8/4/678.full.

8. Anderson, Jane. "What Is Wheat Allergy? Is It the Same as Celiac Disease?" *Verywell* website, updated October 12, 2017, www.verywell.com/what-is-wheat-allergyis-it-the-same-as-celiac-disease-562584.

9. "Strict Adherence for Life Is Essential," www.cureceliacdisease.org/medical-professionals/guide/treatment

10. Takeuchi, H., S. Sekine, K. Kojima, and T. Aoyama. "The Application of Medium-Chain Fatty Acids: Edible Oil with a Suppressing Effect on Body Fat Accumulation." *Asia Pacific Journal of Clinical Nutrition* 17, no. 1 (2008): 320–323. www.ncbi.nlm.nih.gov/pubmed/18296368

11. "Treatment of Celiac Disease." Celiac Disease Center, University of Chicago website, access November 26, 2017, www.cureceliacdisease.org/treatment/.

12. Lanzini, A., F. Lanzarotto, V. Villanacci, A. Mora, S. Bertolazzi, D. Turini, G. Carella, et al. "Complete Recovery of Intestinal Mucosa Occurs Very Rarely in Adult Coeliac Patients Despite Adherence to Gluten-Free Diet." *Alimentary Pharmacology and Therapeutics* 29, no. 12 (2009): 1299–1308, www.ncbi.nlm.nih.gov/pubmed/19302264.

13. Fasano, A. "Leaky Gut and Autoimmune Diseases." *Clinical Reviews in Allergy & Immunology* 42, no. 1 (2012): 71–78, www.ncbi.nlm.nih.gov/pubmed/22109896.

14. Poff, Anglea, Csilla Ari, Thomas N. Seyfried, and Dominic D'Agostino. "The Ketogenic Diet and Hyperbaric Oxygen Therapy Prolong Survival in Mice with Systemic Metastatic Cancer." *PLOS One* 8, no. 6 (2013), http://journals.plos.org/plosone/article?id=10.1371/journal.pone.0065522.

CHAPTER 7

1. Phinney, Stephen. "Does Your Thyroid Need Dietary Carbohydrates?" *Virta* website, May 3, 2017. http://blog.virtahealth.com/does-your-thyroid-need-dietary-carbohydrates/.

2. Rose, C., A. Parker, B. Jefferson, and E. Cartmell. "The Characterization of Feces and Urine: A Review of the Literature to Inform Advanced Treatment Technology." *Critical Reviews in Environmental Science and Technology* 45, no. 17 (2015): 1827–1879, www.ncbi.nlm.nih.gov/pmc/articles/PMC4500995/

3. "The State of American Vacation: How Vacation Became a Casualty of Our Work Culture." *Project: Time Off* website, accessed November 9, 2017, www.projecttimeoff.com/research/state-american-vacation-2016.

CHAPTER 8

1. O'Hearn, Amber. "Ketogenic Diet and Vitamin C: The 101." *BreakNutrition* website, February 21, 2017, http://breaknutrition.com/ketogenic-diet-vitamin-c-101/.

2. "Why Meat Prevents Scurvy." *Autoimmune Thyroid Disease* blog, September 4, 2006, https://autoimmunethyroid.wordpress.com/2006/09/04/why-meat-prevents-scurvy/

3. Matzner, Helmut and Geoffrey H. Bourne. "Die Ascorbinsäure in der Pflanzenzelle. [Vitamin C in the Animal Cell.]" Springer-Verlag, Mar 8, 2013: 1–70.

4. O'Hearn, Amber. "C Is for Carnivore." *Empirica* blog, February 21, 2017, www.empiri.ca/2017/02/c-is-for-carnivore.html.

5. Civitarese, Anthony E., Stacy Carling, Leonie K. Heilbronn, Mathew H. Hulver, Barbara Ukropcova, Walter A. Deutsch, Steven R. Smith, Eric Ravussin, and the CALERIE Pennington Team. "Calorie Restriction Increases Muscle Mitochondrial Biogenesis in Healthy Humans." *PLOS Medicine*, March 6, 2007, http://journals.plos.org/plosmedicine/article?id=10.1371/journal.pmed.0040076.

6. National Park Service. "Brown Bear Frequently Asked Questions." www.nps.gov/katm/learn/photosmultimedia/brown-bear-frequently-asked-questions.htm.

7. Ryan F. Mandelbaum. "Killer Whales Eat Enormous Great White Shark in South Africa." *Gizmodo* website, May 8, 2017, http://gizmodo.com/killer-whales-eat-enormous-great-white-shark-in-south-a-1795016535.

8. Ede, Georgia. "Nightshades." *Diagnosis: Diet* website. www.diagnosisdiet.com/nightshades/

9. Ede, Georgia. "Is Broccoli Good for You?" *Diagnosis: Diet* website, accessed November 9, 2017, www.diagnosisdiet.com/is-broccoli-good-for-you/.

10. Hurrell, Richard F. "Influence of Vegetable Protein Sources on Trace Element and Mineral Bioavailability." *Journal of Nutrition* 133, no. 9 (2003): 2973S–2977S, http://jn.nutrition.org/content/133/9/2973S.long.

11. Ho, Kok-Sun, Charmaine You Mei Tan, Muhd Ashik Mohd Daud, and Francis Seow-Choen. "Stopping or Reducing Dietary Fiber Intake Reduces Constipation and Its Associated Symptoms." *World Journal of Gastroenterology* 18, no. 33 (2012), 4593–4596, www.ncbi.nlm.nih.gov/pmc/articles/PMC3435786/pdf/WJG-18-4593.pdf.

12. Monastrysky, Konstantin. *Fiber Menace: The Truth About the Leading Role of Fiber in Diet Failure, Constipation, Hemorrhoids, Irritable Bowel Syndrome, Ulcerative Colitis, Crohn's Disease, and Colon Cancer.* Ageless Press, 2008.

13. Sinha, Rashmi, Amanda J. Cross, and Barry I. Graubard. "Meat Intake and Mortality: A Prospective Study of Over Half a Million People." *Archives of Internal Medicine* 169, no. 6 (2009): 562–571, http://jamanetwork.com/journals/jamainternalmedicine/fullarticle/414881.

14. "Red Meat Increases Death, Cancer and Heart Risk, Says Study." *BBC News Health* website, March 14, 2012, www.bbc.com/news/health-17345967.

CHAPTER 9

1. Varady, Krista A. and Marc K. Hellerstein. "Alternate-Day Fasting and Chronic Disease Prevention: A Review of Human and Animal Trials." *American Journal of Clinical Nutrition* 86, no. 1 (2007): 7–13, http://ajcn.nutrition.org/content/86/1/7.full

2. Carlson, A. J. and F. Hoelzel. "Apparent Prolongation of the Life Span of Rats by Intermittent Fasting: One Figure." *Journal of Nutrition* 31 (1946): 363–375, www.cabdirect.org/cabdirect/abstract/19461404582.

3. "Timing Meals Later at Night Can Cause Weight Gain and Impair Fat Metabolism." Accessed November 10, 2017, www.sciencedaily.com/releases/2017/06/170602143816.htm.

4. Safide, Fernando, Tanya Dorff, David Quinn, Luigi Fontana, Min Wei, Changhan Lee, Pinchas Cohen, et al. "Fasting and Cancer Treatment in Humans: A Case Series Report." *Aging* 1, no. 12 (2009), 988–1007, www.ncbi.nlm.nih.gov/pmc/articles/PMC2815756/.

CHAPTER 10

1. Nanditha, A., R. C. Ma, A. Ramachandran, C. Snehalatha, J. C. Chan, K. S. Chia, J. E. Shaw, et al. "Diabetes in Asia and the Pacific: Implications for the Global Epidemic." *Diabetes Care* 39, no. 3 (2016), 472–485, www.ncbi.nlm.nih.gov/pubmed/26908931.

2. Blumenthal, James A., Patrick J. Smith, and Benson M. Hoffman. "Is Exercise a Viable Treatment for Depression?" *ACSMs Health Fit J* 16, no. 4 (2012): 14-21, www.ncbi.nlm.nih.gov/pmc/articles/PMC3674785/.

3. Volek, Jeff and Stephen Phinney. *The Art and Science of Low Carbohydrate Living: An Expert Guide to Making the Life-Saving Benefits of Carbohydrate Restriction Sustainable and Enjoyable.* Miami, FL: Beyond Obesity LLC, 2011.

CHAPTER 12

1. Epstein, Leonard, Katelyn Carr, Meghan Cavanaugh, Rocco Paluch, and Mark Bouton. "Long-Term Habituation to Food in Obese and Nonobese Women." *American Journal of Clinical Nutrition* 94, no. 2 (2011), 371–376, http://ajcn.nutrition.org/content/early/2011/05/18/ajcn.110.009035.full.pdf+html.

2. U.S. Department on Health and Human Services Federal Panel on Community Water Fluoridation. "U.S. Public Health Service Recommendation for Fluoride Concentration in Drinking Water for the Prevention of Dental Caries," *Public Health Reports* 130, no. 4 (2015): 318–331, www.ncbi.nlm.nih.gov/pmc/articles/PMC4547570/

INDEX

GRATITUDE

Many people contributed to the writing of this book. First and foremost, I (Craig) want to thank my beautiful wife, Maria. Not only did she write several chapters, but she also took our sons, Micah and Kai, on camping trips to give me time to write. Her drive and strong work ethic help drive me to want to do more, too. She is my inspiration, best friend, business partner, and love of my life. SHMILY

We also want to thank the team at Victory Belt. They have put a ton of effort into this publication. The editors, designers, and entire team did an amazing job. Thank you.

We want to thank Mike Julian for helping us gain a deeper understanding of how our bodies work and for always having the right scientific study for just about any topic. Many others help promote the evidence-based approach to nutrition and are out there trying to help people get healthy and reverse disease processes. Some of the best educators out there are Ivor Cummins (thefatemperor.com), Luis Villasenor (ketogains.com), Tyler Cartwright (ketogains.com), Marty Kendall (optimisingnutrition.com), Dave Feldman (cholesterolcode.com), Ted Naiman (burnfatnotsugar.com), Gabor Erdosi (Facebook group: Lower Insulin), RD Dikeman (Facebook group: Typeonegrit), Robb Wolf (robbwolf.com), and Mark Sisson (marksdailyapple.com). We also want to thank Jimmy Moore for always bringing the leading people in this field to his podcast (livinlavidalowcarb.com) to help spread knowledge. And to the many scientists and doctors promoting a healthy lifestyle, like Dr. Andreas Eenfeldt, Dr. Eric Westman, Dr. Stephen Phinney, Dr. Steve Volek, Dr. Michael Eades, Bill Lagakos, Professor Tim Noakes, Dr. David Ludwig, Gary and Belinda Fettke, Dr. Jeffry Gerber, Dr. Dominic D'Agostino, Dr. Peter Attia, and Dr. William Davis, we appreciate what you do.

We are also thankful for you, the readers and followers of our books and blog. Your support, testimonies, and help spreading the word of health to others enables us to keep going and help more people realize how good their bodies can feel.